BEYOND PSYCHIATRIC EXPERTISE

Publication Number 1063
AMERICAN LECTURE SERIES®

A Monograph in
The BANNERSTONE DIVISION *of*
AMERICAN LECTURES IN BEHAVIORAL SCIENCE AND LAW

Edited by
RALPH SLOVENKO, B.E., LL.B., M.A., Ph.D.
Professor of Law and Psychiatry
Wayne State University Law School
Detroit, Michigan

BEYOND PSYCHIATRIC EXPERTISE

By

BEN BURSTEN, M.D.

Professor
Department of Psychiatry
College of Medicine
The University of Tennessee
Center for the Health Sciences
Memphis, Tennessee

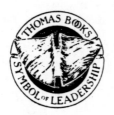

CHARLES C THOMAS • PUBLISHER
Springfield • Illinois • U.S.A.

Published and Distributed Throughout the World by

CHARLES C THOMAS • PUBLISHER
2600 South First Street
Springfield, Illinois 62717

© *1984 by* CHARLES C THOMAS • PUBLISHER

ISBN 0-398-04991-2

Library of Congress Catalog Card Number: 84-2435

With THOMAS BOOKS *careful attention is given to all details of manufacturing and
design. It is the Publisher's desire to present books that are satisfactory as to their physical
qualities and artistic possibilities and appropriate for their particular use.* THOMAS
BOOKS *will be true to those laws of quality that assure a good name and good will.*

Printed in the United States of America
SC R-3

Library of Congress Cataloging in Publication Data

Bursten, Ben.
    Beyond psychiatric expertise.

    (American lecture series. Monograph in American
lectures in behavioral science and law; 1063)
    Bibliography: p.
    Includes index.
    1. Insanity—Jurisprudence—United States.   2. Insane—
Commitment and detention—United States.   3. Forensic
psychiatry—United States.   I. Title.   II. Series.
KF480.B78   1984   346.7301'38   84-2435
ISBN 0-398-04991-2   347.306138

FOREWORD

Questions are daily put: Is one "sick or criminal?" "Sick or praiseworthy?" "Sick or sinful?" "Sick or uneducated?" "Sick or unwise?" "Sick or lazy?" "Sick or malingering?" "Sick or manipulative?" "Sick or merely unpleasant?" "Sick or inexperienced?" These questions lie behind decisionmaking, not only when they are presented directly. They are constantly put to experts in the area of behavior and mental illness. These experts are asked to say whether the behavior of the individual is, fundamentally, a product of mental illness.

We are driven to pose these sick or something-else questions by the powerful emotions of outrage, compassion, or indifference. In the area of psychiatry and law, every test of competency, whether in criminal or civil law, contains a product or "on account of" mental illness question. That is, was a pathological condition, like a human agent, the motivating force behind the act? A person compelled to commit an act (crime or contract) at gunpoint is not held responsible. Likewise, according to the logic, mental illness may threaten a person and force him to do things he would not ordinarily do. Not long ago, the blame was put on the devil or a witch.

The test on criminal responsibility asks about impact of mental illness on cognition or control. For example, the American Law Institute's test, which has been widely adopted, provides that "a person is not responsible for criminal conduct if at the time of such conduct *as a result of mental disease or defect* his capacity either to appreciate the criminality of his conduct or to conform his conduct to the requirements of law is so substantially impaired that he cannot justly be held responsible" (emphasis added). The New Hampshire test of criminal responsibility asks whether the act "was the offspring or product of mental disease." In Edward Oxford's trial in 1840, Lord Denman instructed the jury, "If some controlling disease was, in truth, the acting power within him which he could not resist, then he will not be responsible." Dr. Henry Maudley in 1874 spoke of "morbid impulse" taking despotic possession of the patient and driving him to desperate acts in spite of himself.

Likewise, the test on competency to stand trial asks whether the incompetency was a result of mental illness. The law on civil commitment asks whether on account of mental illness the person is dangerous or in need of care or treatment. The law of contracts provides that certain people ought not to be held responsible for their agreements if they were mentally ill and as a consequence did not know what they were doing. Similarly, the law on testamentary capacity asks whether on account of mental illness the testator realized the nature and extent of his property or the natural objects of his bounty. As one court put it, "The will propounded in this cause . . . being . . . the direct unqualified offspring of that morbid delusion . . . is null and void in law."

There is the idea as well that a positive correlation exists between genius (or at least intellectual eminence) and mental illness. In 1864, Cesare Lombroso published an essay entitled "Genius and Insanity" which was followed by many other writings supporting a connection between psychopathology and creativity. Vincent van Gogh's life has represented to many the destiny of the suffering artist who is marked to endure an unhappy and tragic life as the price of his great genius. Woody Allen, forever in therapy, portrays his psychological conflicts in his films. Kenneth Grahame, author of the classic children's book, "The Wind in the Willows," was subject to obsessive, hysterical and generally abnormal emotional states (as also were Lewis Carroll, Hans Christian Andersen, the Grimm Brothers and Oscar Wilde). A. C. Jacobson in 1926 concluded that while creative individuals may be of insane temperament, their insanity hindered creativity. Lange-Eichbaum in 1932 described geniuses who became psychotic but only after completing their great work (for instance, Baudelaire, Copernicus, Donizetti, Faraday, Kant, Newton, and Stendhal). Other creative people (for instance, Monet, Maupassant, and Rousseau) accomplished great works in the midst of psychosis. Their psychosis and the content of their work remained apart unlike van Gogh, whose psychosis was manifested in his work. Given these personalities and their work, the question has often been put: Would the psychoanalysis of creative people destroy their creativity? The question logically follows the assumption that the creativity is a product or feature of mental illness. Indeed, when a doctor once offered to cure the Norwegian artist Edward Munch of his neuroses he balked, terrified of losing the impetus behind his artistic will.

Social convention brings sick people to doctors; evil people, on the other hand, go to jail. Shall a disruptive person be regarded as sick, sinful, or stupid? Who is properly to make the determination of illness in the first instance? Police officers are daily faced with a "sick or criminal" question in determining whether to take an individual to the hospital or to the police station. A 14-month-old boy was decapitated by his father, Stephen Johnson, who believed his son was Jesus and had to die "for the sins of the world." Should society view him as a criminal or as a patient? What evidence would tilt the decision one way or the other? The lexicon of insanity—not that of evil—was used to describe the Jonestown affair where 909 people, including 262 children, went to their death in a bizarre manner. Their leader, Reverend Jim Jones, was characterized as demented, crazy, paranoid. Why not depraved, cruel, vicious?

The general public assumes that labeling illness is the psychiatrist's role, but people become disenchanted with the conflicting opinions of psychiatrists in particular cases. Dr. Ben Bursten in this book points out the problem is not differing diagnoses but whether there is an illness at all. In equivocal cases, he suggests, the decision to call a cluster of mental characteristics "mental illness" is a matter of policy. The law asks the physician to decide whether there is a "decisive, determinative, causal" relationship between the disease and the act. There may be sick and healthy aspects of mental functioning, however, within the same person. Dr. Bursten argues that there is nothing in a psychiatrist's education or experience which enables him to apportion behavior in this way.

The consequences of a label are immensely important. Which

clusters of mental characteristics are illness and which are not? Sociopathy, at times, was considered an illness. Not long ago, homosexuality was an illness as well; no longer, officially, Whether a cluster of mental characteristics will be considered as mental illness, Dr. Bursten says, will depend on the issue involved and its underlying emotional tensions. One should not expect that mental illness in one area will necessarily be mental illness in another area. In any standard, Dr. Bursten says, the use of terms of degree such as "severe," "substantial," or "serious" to describe a mental illness is at best superfluous and at worst circular.

When are we justified in positing a causal nexus between the behavior and the illness? How do we distinguish between behavior which is a product of illness and that which is a reaction to it? Is the answer anything more than an opinion? What do we mean when we say that certain behavior is a product, or a feature, of mental illness? One could say that mental illness tinges all aspects of the thought processes of the individual, and that every act of the individual is at least partially affected by mental illness. The courts, however, use such phrases as "product of," "causal connection," "because of," "except for," "without which," "but for," "effect of," "result of," "causative factor." The terms, to be sure, are unsatisfying and impenetrable.

Because the label "mentally ill" rests so strongly on questions of policy, why do we spend so much time on these "product of mental illness" problems? Perhaps the need to label is part of human biology and psychology. Certainly society seeks revenge on "bad" persons but apparently not on those who are "sick." Society's label on a particular cluster of mental characteristics corresponds to how it feels about the individual, and society is constantly changing its mind due to competing policy interests. Society's representatives may benefit from psychiatric expertise in determining which cognitive and emotional characteristics are features of a diagnostic category, but it is up to society, through its representatives, to decide whether a behavior is a product of mental illness or not. Psychiatrists may know much about human behavior, but they have no special expertise about how society should be organized. Psychiatry may play a role in pointing out whether a behavior is consistent with that observed in people with the same diagnosis. Ultimately, of course, as Dr. Bursten notes, the jury must decide whom to believe, but the psychiatrist has some expertise in helping to form an opinion.

In this wonderful book, Dr. Bursten engages us in an illuminating discussion of these complex and difficult issues. Written in a lucid style, without jargon or condescension, the book is a pleasure to read, for the quality of the author's thinking, for the perceptiveness of his observations, and for the aptness of his examples. In resolving the "sick or —" questions, expert psychiatric testimony, Dr. Bursten says, is important because the psychiatrist, by virtue of his or her special training, knows which questions to ask the individual in order to illicit important and relevant information regarding his or her mental state. The psychiatrist can formulate the data that are thus collected in terms of the general body of knowledge in the field. It is the application of these data and formulations to the questions asked by society—in society's terms—about sickness, capacities, impairment of free will, and so on, that raises the issue of specific confidence. If the psychiatrist is to be useful to the jury despite the fact that there may be two different frames of reference, Dr. Bursten says, the information from the psychiatric viewpoint must help fuel society's decision-making system. This process of using information from one system to power a different type of system is called "transduction."

The psychiatrist's expertise lies in the medical system of thought; the jury's expertise lies in society's system of thought. In an analogy suggested by Dr. Bursten, consider certain words in one language that have no exact counterpart in another language. Suppose we have a scholar in each language, each of whom knows something about the other's language. We may want to use the services of both in rendering a word or concept from one language to another. Likewise, at trial, we may wish to use the services of both the psychiatrist and the jury.

There are those who state that legal standards, such as the standard of criminal responsibility, derive from a different frame of reference from that usually employed by psychiatrists. If that viewpoint has merit, in order for the psychiatrist to be of assistance to a jury there must be a transduction of information from one frame of reference to the other. At the very least, the jury must make that transduction. It may be valuable, Dr. Bursten says, to provide it with the complementary transduction by the psychiatrist.

Dr. Bursten has a distinguished career in law and psychiatry. He was the major author of the Connecticut confidentiality statute and contributed to legislation on treatment of alcoholics, and on release of information to third-party payers. He is the author of *The Manipulator: A Psychoanalytic View* (Yale University Press, 1973) and numerous articles. He graduated from the University of Vermont with honors in psychology and cum laude from the Yale Medical School and was on the faculty of the Yale Department of Psychiatry from 1964 to 1975. He is a graduate of the Western New England Institute for Psychoanalysis. He is presently Professor in the Department of Psychiatry at the University of Tennessee Center for the Health Sciences.

This is a book of superb scholarly stature.

Ralph Slovenko

INTRODUCTION

During the turbulent 1960s, I was asked to present a series of three lectures about psychoanalysis to an audience of intelligent lay people at a community center. I accepted the invitation with some trepidation, because I knew that some of the topics I would discuss would sound strange and unbelievable to those unfamiliar with the field. I anticipated vigorous and perhaps antagonistic questioning from the audience. However, I was pleasantly surprised at their reaction to the first lecture, which outlined the concepts of repression, the importance of sensuality, and the tendency to repeat experiences of early childhood without being aware of the process. The questions from the floor were thoughtful and showed that the group was eager to learn. There was a similar response to the second lecture, which dealt with psychoanalytic therapeutic technique and the logistics of treatment.

Much to my surprise, the third lecture raised challenges from the audience. This lecture dealt with the application of psychoanalytic insights to the resolution of social problems, and my thesis proposed that this was a very precarious practice. Although psychoanalytic psychiatrists may know a fair amount about human behavior, we have no special expertise about how society should be organized. This view drew protests from several members of the audience. "You mean, with all your knowledge of people, you can't tell us how to improve society?"

I replied that our knowledge about people gave us no special wisdom when judging what would be better or worse for society. They persisted, "But someone must have the answers. If we can't turn to you for guidance, to whom can we turn?"

"That's just the point," I replied. "Why do you expect that I

would know who to turn to any more than you would?" I continued and reminded the audience of the Aesop's fable about the
frogs who wanted a king. They were given a bigger frog to rule
them, but they were dissatisfied. The bigger frog looked just like
themselves—truly he could not be a king. Therefore, the big frog
was removed, and the frogs were given a stork for a ruler. They
were delighted until they realized that their new ruler was eating
them one by one. I cautioned the audience not to let their need for
solutions lead them into uncritical acceptance of what experts
say.

Psychiatrists are idealized by some and scathingly criticized by
others. The admirers believe that the psychological and biological
data we have gathered have greatly enhanced our knowledge of
human nature. They believe we possess the tools to alleviate much
of human suffering, both on an individual and social level. They
sometimes view us with awe, not unmixed with a little fear because we might be able to peek into their own innermost secrets.
But they do turn to us for help and advice.

Critics question whether we have any real data at all. They
point to the abuses of our professional status. They say that under
the mantle of science we wield an inordinate amount of social
power. They are concerned that we drug people into submission,
lull people into conformity, and scare people whose views differ
from our party line, all under the guise of healing.

I believe there is some truth in both positions, but they are
overstated. Psychiatrists do have expertise, based on observation,
experience, and experiment. However, there is much we have to
learn, and our concepts are subject to revision as new data become
available, but there is also much that we know now which we did
not know fifty, twenty-five, or even five years ago. We are putting
our expertise to good use by helping the mentally ill, and there is
every reason to believe that in ten or twenty years, we will have
better expertise.

But we are also human, and we have the same faults as do other
people. Being a psychiatrist does not confer an immunity against
human foibles. And like others who have some expertise, there is
always the temptation to go beyond the limits of that expertise in

an attempt to help, in an attempt to control, or in an attempt to bolster our own self-esteem (and sometimes our pocketbooks) by appearing more knowledgeable than we really are.

There are two ways we psychiatrists can venture beyond our expertise. The first way is that of overpredicting what will happen to the people we study or treat. In many areas, psychiatrists are not very good predictors. Crystal balls are often clouded by insufficient data, inadequate research, and unforseeable outside events. However, while many predictions are beyond our expertise, they are *in principle* within the area of our expertise. If we could obtain sufficient data and do the relevant research, we could improve our record of predictions. Trying to learn which set of facts leads to another set of facts is what psychiatric research is all about, and if our expertise is limited in this area, we must do more research and improve techniques. Applying the known relationships between one set of facts and another is the underlying concept of psychiatric practice (and all medical practice). Unfortunately, sometimes we confuse known facts with facts we wish we knew or believe we know. When this happens, we are beyond our expertise in the area of prediction.

The second way we may go beyond our expertise is to step out of our area altogether. If we psychiatrists claim to be able to advise the city on how to build a bridge over the river, we are not only beyond our predictive expertise but we are out of our area of expertise altogether. Even *in principle* there is no way psychiatric research could help. Building bridges is a matter for engineers. In contrast with the prediction situation, when we are out of our area, we never even will approach the requisite psychiatric expertise.

Of course psychiatrists rarely offer expert opinions on bridges. However, the nature of our work is such that we often are asked to give opinions in a variety of social contexts. As my audience insisted, behavior experts should be able to tell people how to behave. Yet, as I shall show, most of these requests take us out of the psychiatric area and into the areas of ethics and morality. We never, even *in principle,* will have expertise in these areas; they are not our domain.

These, then, are the two ways psychiatrists can and sometimes do go beyond expertise. We predict on the basis of insufficient data, and we go outside of the area of our competence. This book will deal with the second problem. We shall consider why and how psychiatrists go beyond expertise in areas where, even *in principle*, there is no way to establish psychiatric competence. I shall comment on how we can understand this phenomenon and offer some suggestions about how we might attempt to adhere more closely to our own expert area. These issues are complex, and I do not pretend to have resolved them. I hope, at least, that I have faced them.

ACKNOWLEDGMENTS

The primary inspiration for this book came from my patients. They taught me that being a psychiatric patient had impact not only on the mental state but also on social status. Their protests about how others were treating them, and at times how I was treating them, began to penetrate the mantle of professional smugness with which I had cloaked myself. They broadened my outlook and forced me to come to grips with the troubling issues that go with the territory of psychiatry.

The thrust of this book underwent many revisions. It evolved from an emphasis on psychotherapeutic intrusiveness through an attempt to reconcile psychiatry with a deterministic philosophy and emerged in its present form dealing with the problems of exceeding our psychiatric expertise. My wife, Jocelyn, gave me both the time and the attentive ear that I needed to be able to sort out my thoughts. She also endured the unenviable task of being the first critic; she had to tell me when my ideas were senseless or when my prose was unclear. But above all, she gave me the encouragement to write and to rewrite.

Jane Isay, friend and once co-publisher at Basic Books, read several of the early drafts, and with gentle but firm, good humor, she told me to return to the drawing board. Her unique brand of sober encouragement was very helpful.

Dean Nicholas White of the Memphis State Law School graciously allowed me to audit courses in areas germane to my work. Indeed, the ability to use all the library facilities of Memphis State University was indispensible.

I used several people as sounding boards for portions of the manuscript as it was progressing. The comments of Doctors W. Theodore May, John Hutson, and Alan O. Battle and Mr. Robert DeVita were most helpful.

The patience, hard work, and good humor of my secretaries, Beverly Moore in the early phase and Alva Wolfe in the later phase, was above and beyond the call of duty.

All of these people provided suggestions and inspiration, but the responsibility for the ideas and opinions lies solely with me.

CONTENTS

page

Foreword by Ralph Slovenko v

Introduction xi

Chapter

  1. THE SCOPE OF *DURHAM*. 3

  2. MENTAL ILLNESS 23

  3. PRODUCT 45

  4. THE DECISION PROCESS 63

  5. MALINGERING. 83

  6. OUTRAGE–COMPASSION:

      Criminal Responsibility. 94

  7. COMPASSION–INDIFFERENCE:

      The Right to be Left Alone 115

  8. COMPASSION–INDIFFERENCE:

      The Desire to be Designated Sick 142

  9. COMPASSION–INDIFFERENCE:

      Less Coercive Situations 167

 10. SHAM COMPASSION:

      Pseudo-*product* Situations. 198

 11. COMPASSION–COMPASSION:

      The Scope of Psychiatry 220

      INDEX. 251

BEYOND PSYCHIATRIC EXPERTISE

CHAPTER ONE

THE SCOPE OF *DURHAM*

Athirty-year-old man was committed by the court to the psychiatric section of a large Veterans Administration hospital. The man seemed quite calm and rational to the staff. He did not want to be in a hospital; he preferred to be free to lead his vagabond life, roaming all over the South, living with friends and subsisting on checks his mother sent out of a sense of guilt.

Occasionally this man would return home to his upper-middle-class family. They were convinced that he must be sick because he did not join the family business and he could not seem to settle down. They instituted commitment proceedings.

The physician who examined him for the court decided that the man's refusal to work at an available, steady job was a sign of irrationality. No other clinical signs were noted on the commitment papers. Neither the physician nor the attorney appointed to protect the patient's rights, nor the judge felt it was unreasonable to equate refusal to work with mental illness. It took a bit of diplomacy to explain to the judge that while society might prefer to see this man lead a steadier working life, he should not have been confined because mental illness was not the cause of his behavior. What his parents saw as mental illness, this man saw as a life-style.

In the interview, it was noted that he was a very restless person whose wanderings were, at least in part, prompted by a fear of close and socially intimate relationships. He could even be diagnosed—borderline personality disorder. But does applying a label mean that he was mentally ill? Did the man not also have a point? Whatever the reasons, whatever the label, he felt more comfortable living as a wanderer. What was so sick about that? In this instance, the label of mental illness was not applied, and he was released. If he were declared mentally ill, he would have been detained or, at the very least, treatment would have been recommended.

Essentially, the man exhibited a certain behavior cluster— wandering, refusal to work, solitary life, etc. The psychiatric task was to decide if this behavior was a *product of mental illness* or merely representative of a life-style.

Many of the practical decisions that professionals have to make rest on whether a particular behavior is a *product of mental illness.* Indeed, the phrase *product of mental illness* and the concept that underlies it is basic to the practice of psychiatry. It is not basic in a hierarchical sense; not everything stems only from this concept. But it is basic in the sense that so much of what is done requires that a position be taken. If the behavior under scrutiny is a *product of mental illness,* society will act one way; if it is not, society will take a different professional stance.

The phrase *product of mental illness* is known in forensic psychiatry as the *Durham* standard. Monte Durham was a misfit. He did not conform to the Navy when he was seventeen, and he was discharged because of a "profound personality disorder." The next few years were marked by automobile theft, a suicide attempt, passing bad checks, and parole violation. He was shifted from prison to mental hospital, from mental hospital back to prison. He had several court-ordered sanity hearings. Sometimes he was found to have a mental disorder; at other times he was not.

When he was twenty-three years of age, Durham was arrested for housebreaking. At the trial, he pleaded not guilty by reason of insanity. In essence, he admitted doing the offensive act but said he should not be held responsible because he was of unsound mind. The issue before the court was to decide if Monte Durham were sick or criminal. And how could the court decide—what yard-stick could it use? This was settled when Durham appealed his conviction. Judge Bazelon, speaking for D.C. Circuit Court of Appeals (*Durham v. U.S.,* 1954) said that Durham must be found sick "if his unlawful act was the product of mental disease or defect." Disease was defined as a condition capable of improving or deteriorating, while defect was a more static condition. The distinction between disease and defect is not of concern here; for the purpose of this book, the standard shall be modified to read *product of mental illness.*

This standard, this yardstick for making decisions, was not original at the time of *Durham's* appeal in 1954; New Hampshire had a similar standard since 1870 (*State u Pike,* 1870). Nor is it officially in use today; the standard led to such confusion that it was abandoned eighteen years later (*U.S. u Brawner,* 1972). Nonetheless, the ruling of the Court of Appeals received such widespread publicity in the legal and psychiatric literature of the 1950s and 1960s that *product of mental illness* and the concept it stands for is referred to as the *Durham* standard. Monte Durham, a small-time misfit, was awarded a niche in history.

This book deals with the *Durham* standard—*product of mental illness*—but it is not a book primarily about the criminal law. As already demonstrated, this standard is also used in making decisions about whom to commit to mental hospitals. The thesis of this book states that this standard, which Judge Bazelon referred to as simple, has wide application in psychiatry and in decisions society asks psychiatrists to make, is extraordinarily complex and not easily applied because it goes beyond psychiatric expertise, and cannot be avoided in an orderly society.

The standard is applied far beyond the boundaries of the criminal law; it pops up wearing various disguises in many of the everyday activities in which psychiatrists are involved. Yet it is an elusive concept, resting on complicated philosophical points of view rather than scientific facts. When psychiatrists attempt to apply it in decision-making, they often encounter difficulty. Despite these complexities, however, the *Durham* standard is an important vehicle for a smooth-working society. While people will always find it cumbersome and unreliable and they may not feel entirely comfortable with it, the *product of mental illness* standard cannot be abandoned.

The present chapter will deal with the scope of the *Durham* standard and will show how difficult it may be to decide if an act is or is not a *product of mental illness.* Chapters Two and Three will describe the complexities that underlie the standard. These chapters will explain why application of the standard is so difficult. Chapter Four will describe the role that the standard plays in the regulation of society and will offer a framework for understanding how *product of mental illness* is used and how it might be applied. The remaining chapters will illustrate this application in the wide variety of settings in which *product of mental illness* decisions are crucial.

When is society apt to confront the *product of mental illness* issue? Whenever the behavior of a particular individual is deviant (Becker, 1963). Societies tend to value conformity, and those who act differently from most are looked upon with suspicion. If the deviant person seems to cause a disruption or challenges accepted norms, values, or standards of behavior, he or she is given a label, such as "mentally ill, criminal, etc." Labels are not passed out randomly. Society has certain rules governing who is called what, and it follows that how a person is dealt with depends on what he/she is called.

Deviance and normality are not easy to define. Statistical measures may be misleading. If it were possible to count accurately the number of people who have driven automobiles after consuming several drinks, society might be led to classify drinking-and-driving as an accepted standard of behavior. Nevertheless, it goes against the value system.

Essentially, what deviant behavior means in the context of this book is undesirable or unacceptable behavior—the sort of behavior Smart (1961) has termed *dispraiseworthy.* People rarely ask if praiseworthy behavior is a *product of mental illness.* If a person is acting within the framework of society's values, the behavior is accepted at face value. But when people annoy, bother, or harm society, someone may raise the question of whether this behavior is a *product of mental illness.*

The task of distinguishing between praiseworthy and dispraiseworthy behavior is complicated by the fact that the same activities in one social context may pass without question, while in another context, they may be said to be symptomatic of illness. For example, World War II was backed by virtually the entire country. Those who avoided the armed services were seen as deviants and were sometimes included among the mentally ill because of a "lack of sense of responsibility, patriotism, and social obligation" (Lemere and Greenwald, 1943). The Vietnam conflict was much less popular, and those who refused to serve were less likely to be deemed mentally ill.

Even if there is a concensus that a particular behavior is dispraiseworthy, it still may not be viewed as caused by mental illness. Undesirable behavior comes in many forms and gradations. Whereas mental illness is dispraiseworthy, it calls for compassion and treatment. Crime calls for blame and punishment. Sin requires blame, penitence, and prayer. People who make unwise choices need compassion, guidance, and education. Laziness should go unrewarded while manipulativeness should be thwarted. Unpleasant attitudes and behavior merely may need scolding or may require threats and sanctions. Inexperience elicits compassion but calls for guidance, education, or the opportunity to experience.

From the standpoint of the role of practicing psychiatrists and from the many questions asked by society at large, a series of *sick or* _____? questions may be formulated regarding each of the conditions enumerated in the preceding paragraph. Is the person exhibiting the behavior under scrutiny *sick or praiseworthy?, sick or criminal?, sick or sinful?, sick or unwise?, sick or lazy?, sick or manipulative?, Sick or merely unpleasant?, Sick or inexperienced?* Each of these questions requires the psychiatrist, as an expert in the areas of mental and behavioral illness, to determine if the behavior is a product of mental illness. The questions are sometimes asked directly, while at other times psychiatrists hardly are aware that they lie behind their professional activities. As these *sick or* _____? questions are illustrated one by one, the reader will see how wide the scope of *Durham* is, how the *product* issue permeates much of the professional activity, and how it so often confronts questions that may be exceedingly difficult to answer.

Sick or praiseworthy?

In 1978, after several years of hesitation, the American Psychiatric Association focused public opinion on the way in which the Soviet Union uses psychiatrists to stifle dissent. Soviet psychiatry recognizes a mild illness, known as sluggish schizophrenia, which is expressed by withdrawal of interest, rejection of traditions, pessimism, and reformism (Bloch and Reddaway, 1977; Chapter 8). Under this and similar labels, statements critical of the government may be *products of mental illness,* and the dissidents who express such criticism may be confined involuntarily to mental hospitals. In the view of most American observers, the behavior of these dissidents is not a sign of illness but of courage, autonomy, and dignity—praiseworthy, not sick.

The questions of whether certain behavior is a praiseworthy expression of sociopolitical disagreement or a *product of mental illness* have not been confined to the Soviet Union. Several books (Szasz, 1963; Kittrie, 1971; Robitscher, 1980) document psychiatric labelling in the political arena in many countries including America. Chessler (1972) has argued that women seeking liberation, creative assertiveness, and self-expression (praiseworthy behavior when described in these terms) are often diagnosed as ill and maladapted. During the turbulent times of the 1960s, radical psychiatrists (Kunnes, 1970; Hermes, 1971) maintained that by diagnosing deviant behavior as *products of mental illness,* mainstream American psychiatry was being used as a tool in coercing people to submit to and adapt to an oppressive society.

Outside of the political arena, the *sick or praiseworthy?* question may arise in everyday psychiatric practice; for example, in the cyclothymic disorder. People with this type of condition have mood swings. At times, they may be mildly depressed, while during other periods they can be unduly optimistic. During the optimistic periods, they tend to be much more active. They take on new projects often with more enthusiasm than good judgement. One particular man slid into the high part of his cycle with the announcement that he had just met an old acquaintance who had offered him the opportunity to invest in a business venture involving chemical deicers for highways. With an optimism that was as unshakeable as was his pessimism in his low periods, the patient rushed to the bank, withdrew the money, and made the investment. No lawyer was consulted, no credit check was conducted. It seemed to be an impulsive and unwise action. Six months later, the investment paid off handsomely. Was the action the *product of mental illness*—cyclothymic disorder—or was it acutely good business acumen, which the patient could exercise only when he was in an optimistic mood—praiseworthy? Was mental illness causing him to invest impulsively or was it that he was functioning at his best when his spirits were high? He made several other such business deals during the high periods of his cycles, and many of them paid off, and he is now quite a wealthy man. What would have happened if he had been treated as if his behavior were a sign that his illness was worsening? Suppose he had been given medication to calm him down. Would the psychiatrist have blunted his fortune as well as his mood?

Sick or criminal?

The case of Monte Durham illustrates the question of *sick or criminal.* As illustrated in Chapter Six, regardless of the standards of legal insanity that are used, the basic issue comes down to the *Durham* standard: Was the offensive behavior the *product of mental illness?* Even though it is the jury that ultimately makes the decision, the opinion and testimony of psychiatrists has a prominent place in the trial.

Psychiatrists may confront the *sick or criminal?* question outside of the forensic arena also. About 25 percent of the people who ultimately are treated in psychiatric hospitals have been apprehended by police for very minor offenses (Rock et al., 1968, p. 7). Many others are brought to general hospital emergency rooms but are not hospitalized because they are either not sick or not sick enough. The policeman called to the scene of the disturbance makes the initial decision whether the behavior is sick or criminal. If the officer decides the behavior is the *product of mental illness,* he or she will bring the offender to the hospital where it ultimately becomes the psychiatrist's decision to make. If the psychiatrist declares the offender not to be ill, the individual will go to jail rather than to a hospital.

Even within the psychiatric hospital, professionals may be called upon to apply the *Durham* standard to distinguish between sick and criminal. Several years ago, Mr. Johnson was being treated on a psychiatric ward. He had come in with a moderate depression, which was diagnosed as mental illness. As psychiatrists and staff got to know him, they became aware of his very difficult family situation, and offered to help him and his wife work things out. Mr. Johnson had quite a temper, which would flare up at times, and which, at other times, would subside into a smouldering resentment. While some of the dynamics underlying this behavior could be understood, the doctors viewed the temper not as a *product of mental illness* but as an unpleasant attitude.

One day, after telephoning an acquaintance in a distant city, Mr. Johnson became enraged claiming that the acquaintance had cheated him out of some money. He stated that he had a gun in his car and he was going to drive to the acquaintance's city to kill him. Although the staff attempted to talk him out of it, he was adamant. He was strong, and while he could have been restrained, there would have been quite a struggle. Legally, he could have been declared sick—insane and dangerous, not responsible for his action—and he could have been detained. But his temper was not viewed as the *product of mental illness*. He was informed that he was not insane and if he chose to shoot someone, he should be held criminally responsible. He was also told that if he left, the police would be notified since the matter was no longer medical—it had become a legal matter.

Mr. Johnson did leave and the police were called to inform them about the situation. A few hours later, the police called to say that they had apprehended Mr. Johnson, and indeed, he did have a gun in his car. The police wanted to know what to do with the patient, but the psychiatrists involved felt it was a legal matter. The hospital staff, of course, was still willing to help Mr. Johnson with his family situation, but the matter of the intended shooting was a legal, not a medical question. The police, however, chose to view it differently and they returned him to the hospital without pressing charges.

Sick or sinful?

It is not uncommon for some people with a strong religious viewpoint to characterize as sinful behavior that which some psychiatrists see as a *product of mental illness* (Runions, 1975). Christian psychiatrists (usually biblical literalists, not to be confused as a group with all psychiatrists who may attend a Christian church of any denomination) speak of three levels—the physical, the psychological, and the spiritual. As Minirth (1977) says,

Perhaps the problem did not start on a physical or psychological level, but on a spiritual level. For example, the individual may have chosen to sin and commit adultery. His guilt feelings may lead to anxiety and then to an ulcer. . . .

. . . how can a counselor treat a spiritual problem if he uses only psychological and physical therapies? *Man is a whole, comprised of more than one part, and he must be treated as such* (Minirth's italics).

In this view, the ulcer is seen as the *product of mental illness* — the guilt, but the guilt is seen as the product of sin — adultery. The therapeutic program will depend on whether the adulterous behavior is interpreted as sick or sinful. The Christian psychiatrist might pray with the patient and urge him or her to accept Christ in order to have the willpower necessary to resist the temptation of further sin.

In psychotherapy, patients with a biblical-literalist frame of reference frequently view certain thoughts or impulses as sinful. The psychiatrist, on the other hand, might offer a more naturalistic explanation. While the conflict of viewpoints often arises over sexual urges, it may appear in other areas as well. For example, certain compulsive patients have a smouldering, underlying anger toward parents, siblings, etc. They may repress this anger and cover it with a need to ingratiate themselves with others — to be perfectionistic and pleasing. The anger must be controlled, kept back — even if it means that the patient cannot let go enough to have any fun at all. During the course of psychotherapy as the patient begins to become aware of the underlying anger, he or she may balk. Patients may say, "I don't want to go into this area; I don't want to be angry because it is un-Christian to hate." To them, the anger is a product of sin, not a product of their inhibition that has prevented them from coming to grips with the emotion.

Sick or unwise?

The *sick or unwise?* question is likely to arise in several types of settings. The practicing psychiatrist must confront it, the psychiatric consultant frequently is asked to decide the question, and the forensic psychiatrist often becomes involved in this type of *product* issue.

Every time a patient is taken into treatment, his or her presenting behavior is labeled tacitly as a *product of mental illness*. This usually poses no significant problem, unless the patient comes unwillingly—through legal compulsion, through social pressure of relatives or friends, or as a child brought by concerned parents. When the prospective patient does not want a psychiatrist to interfere in his or her life, as in the case of the man committed because of his vagabond life-style, the *sick or unwise?* question may leap to the forefront and need to be faced directly.

The issue also arises when patients have been committed to a psychiatric hospital. Recent "right to refuse treatment" cases (*Rennie v Klein*, 1981; *Rogers v Okin*, 1980) have been concerned with just how far psychiatrists can go in forcing committed patients to take medication against their will. There may be various reasons that hospitalized patients will refuse medication. They may resent their hospitalization. They may feel that they are being medicated not so much for illness, but because the staff wants a quiet ward—a system of control rather than treatment. They may be frightened about possible long-term, debilitating side effects. They may believe they are not ill, or that they will not get worse without medicine. They may have delusions that the medicine is a trick, or they may have hallucinations warning them not to cooperate. They may be too confused to weigh the risks and benefits in a coherent manner. Or they may enjoy the symptoms of their illness, such as a feeling of elation, great power, and energy, which they do not want to surrender. The courts generally have taken the position that, except for emergency situations with imminent danger, a competent patient may refuse medication. And when is a patient incompetent? When his or her refusal of medication is not a reasoned decision—when it is a *product of mental illness.* The decision maker must decide if this refusal is sick or merely unwise.

This decision is not always easy. For example, a bright but psychotic executive secretary sometimes, despite her medications, became delusional. She would begin to think that all food that was neither black or white was poisonous. The pills were orange, so she threw them down the toilet. A discussion of her reasons left little doubt that the action was a *product of mental illness.* But there were other times when she was not delusional. Sometimes, even when her thoughts were not disordered, she would become frightened as she remembered her sicker periods. She used the defense mechanism of denial: "I do not have an illness, I do not have an illness. Then why take pills?" Or, alternatively, "If I take the pills, it means I do have the dreaded illness." Before these thoughts are dismissed as the *product of mental illness*—the psychotic productions of a seriously disturbed person—it should be noted that many people will not go to a hospital because people die there. Or they will not go to a doctor because "he or she may find out I'm sick." And how many believers in scientific, statistical data continue to smoke cigarettes despite the mounting evidence of health hazards, because of an inner conviction that "It won't (can't) happen to me?" Was the executive secretary *sick or unwise?*

The psychiatrist who consults on the medical and surgical services of a general hospital may confront similar problems. For example, an elderly lady who has developed gangrene in her legs may require amputation in order to prevent the condition from spreading to the point where it will be life threatening. She may refuse to sign an operation consent form. The vascular surgeon, observing that the patient becomes a bit confused and disoriented, especially at night, may ask for a psychiatric consultation. The psychiatrist may learn that the patient bases her decision to refuse the operation on the belief that the doctor is in league with her son. The plan is to kill her during surgery in order that the son may get the inheritance. Professionals would probably conclude that her decision is a *product of mental illness.* They would convey that opinion to a judge who might declare her incompetent and appoint a guardian for her.

However, what if she says she does not want the operation because she would rather die than spend the rest of her life without her legs? Suppose she has adequate financial resources to live fairly comfortably, and she can afford the assistance she would need after the operation. But she is a proud woman who puts great stock in being independent. She may be confused at times, but she is clear about her pride and her position. Is her refusal a *product of mental illness*—the result of an intense narcissism and the stubbornness and rigidity that sometimes accompanies advancing age? Is this *sick or unwise?*

Psychiatrists who consult with social agencies, schools, governmental units, etc. frequently are asked for an opinion (often off the record) about whether someone is acting irrationally or merely foolishly. And think of the heavy weight of the *sick or unwise?* decision when the behavior under scrutiny is that of the President of the United States (Robitscher, 1980, pp. 344ff.).

In the area of forensic psychiatry, the *sick or unwise?* issue usually centers around competence. Does the person have the capacity to make a contract or to get married? If a will looks foolish to relatives who have been cut off from an inheritance, was it, perhaps, the product of an unsound mind? And in custody battles, the difference between an unwise parent and a mentally ill one may carry great weight.

Sick or lazy?/Sick or manipulative?

The *sick or lazy?* and the *sick or manipulative?* questions often go together because the lazy person frequently will pretend to be sick in order to avoid work. Psychiatrists working in schools and colleges often confront this issue. Did the student miss the examination or perform poorly during the previous semester because he or she was too lazy to do the work or was he or she under such severe emotional stress that the lack of studying ought to be considered a *product of mental illness,* albeit a mild one? Psychiatrists working in the armed forces, in industry, or in prisons confront similar situations.

Disability examinations offer a good example of the type of situation where these two questions are coupled. The worker claims to be sick and unable to work. He or she feels entitled to receive Social Security benefits. According to the Social Security Administration (20 CFR 404.900), if the applicant claims that the disability is the *product of mental illness,* the restriction in his or her work functioning must be based on "medical evidence consisting of demonstrable clinical signs. . . . " If the patient says he or she is hearing voices and believes that ghosts are sapping his or her strength making him or her too weak to work, this report becomes medical evidence only if it is reasonably certain the individual is not faking. The distinction between sickness on the one hand and laziness and manipulation on the other may be difficult to make.

One thing that complicates the disability situation is the rewards for faking can be very great. For example, the *product* question *sick or greedy?* might have been posed. And, indeed, there are situations where manipulativeness comes uncoupled from laziness and greed is pursued with vigor. For example, after a severe automobile accident, a person may not wish to stop working. Nonetheless, the individual may complain of tension, sleep difficulty, anxiety, and a host of other problems. He or she may be suing the driver of the other vehicle for damages. If the doctors and the courts decide these complaints are genuine, the product of a posttraumatic stress disorder, the litigant will be compensated. If they decide the individual was faking or manipulating, no money will be awarded.

Another area where the *Durham* standard focuses on *sick or manipulative?* is that of psychotherapy. Some psychiatrists view all behavior that is not demonstrably, biologically driven as manipulative. Following Szasz (1961), they declare that patients adopt a posture of illness with the purpose of influencing others to act and to react in certain ways. In essence, what appears as mental illness is really manipulation. These psychiatrists have decided that no behavior is a *product of mental illness.* This decision may have a significant impact on how they conduct psychotherapy (a strange response to a nonill person). Often they view the therapeutic encounter as a chess game that requires the therapist to develop a strategy to counter the manipulative strategy of the opponent—the client or patient. (For a more detailed description of this viewpoint, see Bursten, 1973a, Chapters 2 and 13.) Whether psychiatrists view their patients' behavior as sick or manipulative has considerable influence on the approach taken in the consulting room.

Sick or merely unpleasant?

Whereas the manipulative person claims he or she is entitled to something because of illness, the unpleasant person usually wants to be left alone and resents being seen as sick. The behavior under scrutiny may be merely annoying, it may be disruptive, or it may be felt to be dangerous almost to the point of being criminal. Society demands disciplinary action, and sometimes the psychiatrist is called to settle the matter. The *sick or merely unpleasant?* issue can arise both when the psychiatrist is acting as a consultant to others and in course of general psychiatric practice.

The medical director of a large federal facility asked to have evaluated one of the employees, Mr. Donovan, to see if he had a psychiatric disability that would render him medically unfit to continue work. Mr. Donovan came to see the psychiatrist under protest; he was convinced that the evaluation was part of his supervisor's scheme to get him fired.

The employee said he had worked for this agency for six years and he had an excellent work record. He was a man of very high principles, and he believed in "a good day's work for a day's pay, which is more than you can say for a lot of people in my office." He was particularly irritated with the morals and standards of his supervisor, who not only took too much time off, but who was using government office machines to conduct his own private business on the side. As if that were not indignity enough, on occasion the supervisor had asked Mr. Donovan to perform certain computer tasks for his business on government computers on government time. Mr. Donovan was not able merely to decline; he had to argue and lecture the supervisor. He became openly contemptuous. The boss, who was generally easygoing, might have let the matter drop, but to Mr. Donovan this was a matter of principle, and his supervisor's cheating gnawed at him. While his work performance remained at its usual high level, Mr. Donovan's remarks and nasty glances made life intolerable for his boss.

Mr. Donovan contended that the government had no grounds on which to fire him and that the supervisor hoped to get him declared medically unfit in order to get rid of him. Although the supervisor did not mention that he was using government equipment for his private business, his description of Mr. Donovan's activities at work generally agreed with what the employee had said. Mr. Donovan did do his work, but his attitude was so negative, so poor, that it was interfering with morale. The issue to consider, then, was whether the employee's behavior was a *product of mental illness* or an irritating attitude. Was it *sick or merely unpleasant?* If it was the former, he would be let go; if the latter, they probably would not risk firing Mr. Donovan because he was the type who would sue.

While Mr. Donovan was generally suspicious of people, overly ready to ferret out injustices, and exceedingly critical of those who failed to live up to his own rather inflexible moral standards, his grip on reality was firm and his thinking processes showed no gross distortions. It could be predicted with reasonable certainty that with this type of personality, he would discover big or little injustices wherever he worked and that he was highly likely to be involved in arguments and disputes.

Was he *sick or merely unpleasant?* Once again, just because there is a diagnostic label for this kind of person, should it be reported to the medical director that Mr. Donovan was sick and medically unfit to work? The decision was made to describe him as provocative. To take the position that whether such an unpleasant man should continue to work would have to be an administrative rather than a medical decision.

The attempt to use the psychiatric consultant to solve disciplinary problems is a common occurrence in the general hospital setting. People with medical and surgical illnesses can be psychiatrically ill simultaneously. Indeed, sometimes the mental illness results from the disturbances in body chemistry, which is a feature of the medical illness. Sometimes it may be a reaction to the medicine the patient is receiving. But there are other situations, such as the cantankerous patient with a heart attack or the pseudoindependent patient whose intolerance of being helpless leads him or her to bicker and fight with the staff. Are these behaviors the *product of mental illness?* Are they *sick or merely unpleasant?*

Many nonpsychiatric physicians expect their patients to be as docile as laboratory animals; many nurses demand quiet and cooperation from their patients. When these individuals do not fit the mold of the good and cooperative patient, when their behavior threatens the peace and order of the ward, the staff needs a disciplinarian. Sometimes the psychiatrist is called. Docility is also expected of school children. Children may misbehave for a variety of reasons—a disturbed home situation, an impossibly rigid and demanding teacher, a grade placement that is too high or too low, poor nutrition, poor training that has left them undersocialized, emotional problems such as shame or inferiority feelings, learning disabilities, brain dysfunction, etc. The prime causes of the restless behavior may lie within the child or outside of the child. When the behavior is viewed as unpleasant, at the very least external causes should be considered. When the behavior is viewed as sick, the child becomes the object to be changed.

Although many childhood disciplinary problems are not the result of mental illness, the hyperkinetic syndrome is one disorder that seems to result from a brain dysfunction. It prevents the child from adequately integrating stimuli. Hyperkinetic children have very short attention spans, are terribly distractable, have unusual sleep patterns, and cause social havoc at home and in school. Methylphenidate hydrochloride seems to improve the integrating power of these children's brains and therefore calms them down. It is much easier to administer this medication to children than to attend to the noxious social situations arising both in and out of school. And so, it is not surprising that the medicine quickly gained popularity in the 1970s and more and more children who were nuisances in school were diagnosed as hyperkinetic (Schrag and Divosky, 1975). Some probably were; many probably were not (Greenberg, et al., 1972). When does a school discipline problem become a psychiatric problem — that is, the *product of mental illness?*

Medications are used with mentally retarded people who are difficult to manage either at home or in institutions. These drugs may be used to calm down individuals who are too sexually active, too angry, too disobedient, etc. How much sexual activity, anger, or disobedience is too much? Is the psychiatrist being used as doctor or disciplinarian? Is the patient's behavior unpleasant or the *product of mental illness?* Often it may be difficult to decide.

Disciplinary problems may arise not only in the consultation setting, but in the general practice of psychiatry as well. No patient is psychotic 100 percent of the time. When they disturb the peace and quiet of the hospital ward, it is all too easy to say that their behavior is a *product of mental illness* and to medicate them. Often this is true. But sometimes the patients more properly may be called unpleasant rather than sick. Especially in overcrowded and understaffed wards, patients may become irritable, obstinate, anxious, restless, etc., not because they are sick but because they are human. Often the line of least resistance (and minimal cost) is to sedate these people with medication on the grounds of mental illness. As one beleaguered psychiatrist said recently, "I'd trade half of the medicine on the unit for one television set." And yet, when the ward doctor receives the telephone call from the nurse that a patient is excited and agitated, it may be difficult to determine if the behavior is the *product of mental illness.*

Sick or inexperienced?

In the discussion of *sick or manipulative?*, some psychotherapists, view all behavior as manipulative and engage in a kind of therapeutic chess game in order to outwit their patients. In other words, how the psychiatrist views the behavior that brings the patient to the consulting room in the first place strongly will influence his or her psychotherapeutic stance. For some psychiatrists, the psychotherapeutic issue is not *sick or manipulative?* but *sick or inexperienced?* Except for behavior that has striking biological input, such as senile dementias, some psychiatrists and other psychotherapists view patients' concerns and maladaptations not as *products of mental illness* but as problems of living. According to these practitioners, these patients, often called *clients* to get away from the medical connotation, do not need diagnosis and treatment. They may need counselling, guidance, training, practice, education, or the opportunity to experience their inner selves and to grow. The assumption behind this point of view is that there is no disorder underlying the behavior under scrutiny; there is instead the need for further development. Nothing is actually wrong, but an inner potential has been blocked or diverted. Various approaches that rest on this assumption and point of view are described by Rychlak (1973). The term *inexperience,* is used to refer to a state where there is no *mal*function but a *lack* of *optimal* functioning.

Therapists who resolve the *product* issue in terms of inexperience rather than sickness do not look for causes or pathological processes that must be cured and removed in order for healing to occur. For example, May argued against Freud's concept of psychopathology.

> Freud is seduced by the handy, tangible systematization of natural science; and he uses it as a procrustean bed on which he lays the human personality and finds it to fit . . .

If such a determinism is accepted, human responsibility is destroyed. . . .
What of purpose and freedom and creative decurum on the part of the
individual? (May, 1939, p. 48ff)

May was saying that the framework of natural science is too
confining for the study and treatment of the human personality
and behavior. Even though it might be possible to view behavior as a product of illness, it is inappropriate because the
frame of reference does not allow for growth and development of
responsibility, freedom, purpose, and creativity.

The *sick or inexperienced?* question goes far beyond any particular psychiatrist's view of human behavior and psychotherapy. It
reaches into the very definition of what psychiatry is and what
psychiatrists should and should not deal with. There have been
some who have argued that psychiatrists have taken on too many
areas (Torrey, 1974; Siegler and Osmond, 1974; Ludwig and Othmer,
1977). They maintain that it is possible to distinguish between
behavior, which is a *product of mental illness* and that which is a
problem of living—the concept that would fall into the category of
problem of inexperience. According to these writers, psychiatry,
being a medical specialty, should deal only with the former, while
problems of living should be handled by other specialists with a
nonmedical orientation. Thus, whether any particular behavior is
considered a *product of mental illness* determines if it is a fit area for
psychiatric involvement altogether. Or, conversely, since psychiatry is defined in great measure by what psychiatrists do, the
definition and extent of the field is determined by which people
with deviant behavior are seen as sick and which are seen as
inexperienced.

Other psychiatrists (Astrachan et al., 1976; Adler, 1981) have
taken a middle course. They, too, seem to separate illness from
problems of living, but they maintain that the psychiatrist's tasks
are not necessarily confined to the medical area. Thus, they propose four psychiatric tasks—the medical, the rehabilitative (brought
into play when there is no illness or when the disease is arrested or
cured), the societal–legal (the interface between psychiatrists and
the demand of society that its deviants be controlled), and the
educative–developmental (growth of the individual in order that
he or she may realize his or her potential).

But the distinction between illness and problems of living—between sick and inexperience—is not that easily made, and there are those psychiatrists (Engel, 1979, Bursten, 1979a) who caution against too narrow a definition of what is properly a medical function. Stress, for example, clearly can arise in the context of living situations. Yet it has a significant role in a variety of medical illnesses. Is stress a medical problem? Are behaviors induced by stress the *product of mental illness* or inexperience? Are such behaviors and the situations that bring them about the proper domain of psychiatry?

This problem of role and task definition concerns not only how psychiatrists see themselves—their professional identity, but also how others see them and what they do. As medical treatment is increasingly paid for by third parties, whether private insurance companies or government, there is a need to establish that such interventions are medically necessary. With the tightening of economic conditions, third party payers are more and more reluctant to foot the bill for the resolution of problems of living. For them, too, the question of whether the behavior under scrutiny (and under the psychiatrist's care) is a *product of mental illness* is very important. They may be willing to insure against sickness but not inexperience.

Likewise, the research enterprise of the psychiatry profession can be influenced significantly by the *sick or inexperienced?* question. In any era, what is discovered is significantly dependent on cultural values (Mannheim, 1952). The behaviors that are considered *products of mental illness* are more likely to be investigated. Society is more likely to fund research into those behavior clusters that are labeled sick than those that are called problems of living. Even the research techniques used and the types of data from which conclusions are drawn can be influenced by this question. The technological explosion of the latter half of the twentieth century has started to bear significant fruit and gives enormous promise in psychiatric research. Will this lead to a situation in which only those behaviors that can be measured technologically, behaviors which have biological markers, will be called legitimate mental illnesses? Will introspective behavior—reports of thoughts and feelings—take a back seat in the research arena because they may have been defined out of the illness category?

What is seen when the *Durham* standard—the *product of mental illness*—is translated into a series of *sick or* _____*?* questions and especially when *sick or inexperienced?* is considered is that the standard touches on all psychiatric activity and reaches into the core of psychiatric professional identity. *Durham* has a very wide scope indeed.

Monte Durham, the small-time bad check passer and housebreaker, was a misfit, and misfits are what psychiatry is concerned with. But psychiatrists do not deal with all misfits—just the ones whose behavior is considered a *product of mental illness.* The simple standard that the court put forth to distinguish between sick and criminal is really a basic conundrum to be faced when psychiatrists attempt to distinguish between sick and anything. However, this is not simple at all, nor can it be avoided. Psychiatry, by its very nature, is involved in tough decisions that a society needs to have made. This book will examine those questions and the process by which they are resolved.

CHAPTER TWO

MENTAL ILLNESS

In order to apply the *Durham* standard—*product of mental illness*—to any decision-making situation, mental illness must first be defined and recognized. The term and the concept it represents can be quite slippery. Even if a diagnostic label is put on a behavior cluster, such as *borderline personality disorder* to label the young wanderer who refused to work in Chapter One, it may still be difficult to decide whether to call this cluster a mental illness.

This difficulty is well illustrated by what has been called one of the classic fiascos in psychiatry. The setting was St. Elizabeths Hospital in Washington, D.C. and the principals were Doctors Overholser and Duval. Dr. Winfred Overholser, the hospital superintendent, had been president of the American Psychiatric Association in 1947 and 1948. He was a professor of psychiatry at George Washington University School of Medicine. In 1952, he received the Isaac Ray Award for the outstanding contribution to forensic psychiatry. Dr. Addison Duval, the assistant superintendent was also a professor at George Washington University. He was the Vice President of the American Psychiatric Association in 1964 and later became Commissioner of Mental Health of the State of Georgia. Both doctors were respected highly. They were not intemperate men or radical thinkers; they were very sober and thoughtful men who were rooted solidly within the mainstream of the profession.

The diagnostic category that was the subject of this fiasco was that of sociopathy, or, as it is currently called, antisocial personality. This has always been a troublesome diagnosis because people so labelled generally can think rationally and are free of delusions and hallucinations. First and foremost, sociopathic people have a blatant disregard for the norms, values, and laws of society. They are very self-centered. They tend to lie and deceive other people. They seem to suffer very little guilt or remorse. The question was whether persons exhibiting these characteristics are mentally ill.

In 1952, the American Psychiatric Association (APA) published its first official *Diagnostic and Statistical Manual of Mental Disorders* ([DSM I], APA, 1952). It listed sociopathic personality as a mental illness. However, shortly after the *Durham* decision in 1954, mental hospital superintendents became concerned that large numbers of sociopathic criminals would be considered mentally ill and thus found not guilty by reason of insanity. Instead of being sent to prison, they would go to mental hospitals. Physicians in mental hospitals generally do not like to treat sociopathic persons for several reasons. First, there is no firm treatment modality for this condition. Second, these people are liars, cheaters, and deceivers. They often cause a great deal of disruption on the hospital ward. They prey on vulnerable patients whose thinking processes are dulled or confused by other mental conditions. They irritate staff and fail to cooperate with rules. Clearly, something had to be done to prevent an anticipated influx of such people.

Dr. Duval explained what happened (*United States v. Leach,* 1957).

> Late in 1954, after the *Durham* decision, we had a staff meeting [at St. Elizabeths Hospital] at which the psychiatrists discussed what should be the uniform, if possible, type of name which we would give to this particular group of cases, known as sociopathic personality disturbance, namely whether we would report them as with mental disorder or without mental disorder. . . .
>   The decision at that time was that in the agreed-upon consensus of our psychiatric staff this group of individuals so classified would be considered without mental disorder. . . .

Thus, in 1954, by a decision made at a staff meeting, sociopathic people lost their status as mentally ill.

Three years later, Doctors Overholser and Duval reversed their opinion. Administratively, they decided that as of November 18, 1957 in St. Elizabeths Hospital, a sociopathic personality would be considered a mental illness. And in 1962, Dr. Overholser (1962) reaffirmed this decision, "The sociopath . . . is decidedly a mentally sick man."

Is sociopathy a mental illness? It was in 1953; it was not in 1954; it was in 1957, and once again in 1962. Now you see it, now you don't.

One sociopathic man, Mr. Comer Blocker, complained that on October 22, 1957, at the time of his first trial, sociopathic personality was not a mental disease. However, a few weeks later, it became a mental illness. Because of this new medical evidence, he was given a new trial (*Blocker u United States*, 1959).

What was this new medical evidence? There were no new empirical facts that had been discovered. There were no new laboratory findings nor were there large-scale community statistical studies of course and outcome. This "new medical evidence" was that Dr. Duval and Dr. Overholser had changed the rules; they were prepared to testify that sociopathy was, indeed, a mental illness. This illness was created (or rather re-created) in conference as *a matter of policy.* The whole scenario did, indeed, seem like a fiasco, although in retrospect it was not as much of a farce as it appeared to be.

If the Overholser-Duval policy decision was a fiasco, it does not stand alone. Such conditions as alcoholism and homosexuality have also changed with regard to acceptance versus being a mental illness. As Robtischer (1980, pp. 162 ff.) pointed out, these changes have not been the result of significant new empirical evidence but rather the result of shifts in policy. They differ from the Overholser-Duval episode largely because the changes have been made by more than two people; indeed, they have been endorsed by a very significant segment of the psychiatric profession. In addition, these were not sudden single conference decisions, but rather were the result of evolution, discussion, and relatively slower acceptance.

Alcoholism used to be regarded, at best, as a bad habit. Although there were always some in the psychiatry field who maintained that there is a biologically driven compulsion behind alcoholism which seemed to qualify it for the label illness, many professionals treated alcoholics as if they were morally despicable. Nonetheless, when alcoholism became recognized as a national problem and there were monies available for research and hospitalization, there was a gradual change in attitude toward accepting alcoholism as a legitimate illness that should be both investigated and treated. In all fairness, it should be recorded that there have been slow and steady advances pointing toward some biochemical and genetic underpinnings of this condition. However, it was not these new bits of evidence that startled doctors and scientists into the sudden recognition of alcoholism as an illness; instead, it was a policy decision that was guided in great measure by the availability of economic resources.

The policy change that removed homosexuality from the illness category is well described by Robtischer (1980, pp. 170 ff.). In DSM II (1968), homosexuality was categorized as a disease. However, during the late 1960s and early 1970s, gay activists were advancing the notion that homosexuality was a sexual orientation—a way of life—and not an illness. They forcefully intruded into several professional meetings and engaged psychiatrists in vigorous debate. In the social climate of protest against the arbitrary repression of dissidents and harmless deviants, in 1973, the Board of Trustees of the American Psychiatric Association decided homosexuality was not a disease. This decision subsequently was ratified by 58 percent of the voting members of the association. Thus, as a matter of policy, a condition that previously had been considered pathological was no longer an illness. Again, there were no significant empirical findings to support this change other than the fact that cultural values in general had shifted. Presently there are still a significant number of psychiatrists who disagree with the decision. They continue to consider homosexuality an illness and feel that the American Psychiatric Association's decision was a fiasco.

The issue must be clear. The question is not whether psychiatrists are able to agree on any particular diagnosis. The problem is not that some psychiatrists may diagnose a person as having one illness while other psychiatrists may say the individual has a different illness. The problem is that given a particular diagnostic category, there may be disagreement about whether the behaviors it connotes constitute an illness at all.

How does a psychiatrist decide whether the cluster of characteristics constitutes an illness? Probably the first criterion that occurs is suffering. Pain, discomfort, malaise, and distress would seem to be the hallmarks of sickness.

However, there are many conditions usually considered to be

illness that are not accompanied by suffering. The early stages of cancer may be undetected by the individual. Serious hypertension may be silent for many years. In the realm of mental illness (a concept to be dealt with shortly), mania often is characterized by an elated feeling that things were never quite so good as they are now. Deliria and dementias, those many dysfunctions of the brain due to the insults of alcohol, drugs, trauma, degeneration of parts of the nervous system, etc., may all be marked by a surprising lack of serious subjective discomfort, particularly in view of the often high degree of impairment involved. On the other hand, any psychiatrist will recognize that there are conditions where the pain and suffering are inaccurate signals. Psychogenic pain, for example the experience of a painful back when there is no pathology in the back, has been called a disease by some and has been called a nondisease by others. Worrying, obsessive brooding, fear, and minor anxieties, are all discomforts, yet they are not accepted universally as necessarily being indicators of sickness. Thus, while suffering is important as a signal that something is wrong, it cannot be said to be a reliable criterion of illness.

A second common definition of illness is the absence of health. This approach attempts to arrive at a consensus about what constitutes normal functioning (Jahoda, 1958; Offer and Sabshin, 1980); when this is found to be lacking, the person is considered to be sick. However, particularly in the realm of human behavior, there is such a wide variation that it is probably impossible even to approach a consensus on what is normal. Most definitions seem to describe adaptedness (which may be a vigorous way of coping with what society has to offer or may be a timid or mindless knuckling under) or someone's version of the ideal person (which makes everyone *sick*).

Despite these difficulties, illness must be defined if the *product of mental illness* standard in decision-making is to be used. Scholars such as Parsons (1951, Chapter 10), Friedson (1970), and Wing (1978), have considered the definition of health and illness. Following their contributions, illness reasonably can be defined by six criteria.

1. There is a cluster of characteristics.
2. This cluster is undesirable.

3. This cluster takes a natural course and there is presumed to be a rational explanation for this course in terms of antecedents and outcome.
4. This cluster has a predominately biological process as its focus.
5. This cluster has a predominately individual rather than social focus.
6. This cluster is beyond the individual's control; he or she cannot choose to change the characteristics by willpower.

THE CLUSTER OF CHARACTERISTICS

The cluster of characteristics serves to identify a given condition. Fever, cough, weakness and night sweats, the appearance of certain bacteria on microscopic examination of sputum, certain types of white patches seen on the X rays of the lungs, etc. are a cluster of characteristics that identify tuberculosis. Litigiousness, argumentativeness, mistrustfulness, inability to form warm relationships, logical but quibbling patterns of thinking, etc. are a cluster of characteristics that identify a paranoid personality. Whether either or both of these clusters are called illness depends on whether the other four criteria are met. The clusters identify the conditions and differentiate them from each other.

Mental illness would be identified by a cluster of mental characteristics. These characteristics are thoughts, feelings, and behavior. While most people would agree that thoughts and feelings are mental qualities, behavior seems so objective, so physical, that it appears to be out of place with the other two. However, behavior does not refer to mere movement; if a man falls off a scaffold, the fact that he is moving rapidly downward does not indicate behavior. But if he yells, extends his arms and legs to break his fall, or shuts his eyes, these are behaviors because they occur in a personal context and have meaning (thoughts and feelings) to the individual.

Most observable bodily events have meaning to the individual. Aches and pains, skin yellow with jaundice, deformity of the hip, etc. cannot help but be personally significant. Yet the usual reactions to these afflictions are not considered to be mental illness. Only when the cluster of mental characteristics achieves a certain prominance are they focussed on.

Traditionally, these characteristics have been used to indicate mental illness in two settings. First, clusters in which the most prominent characteristics are thoughts, feelings and behavior are called mental illness. Thus, people with schizophrenia capture attention because their thinking is distorted, they cannot integrate their feelings with their actual situation, and they behave oddly.

Psychiatric research seems to be on the threshold of discovering the neurochemical underpinnings of schizophrenia. With discoveries such as these, will schizophrenia no longer be a mental illness? Will it be a neurological or physical illness? Some psychiatrists (Szasz, 1974, Chapter 2; Torrey, 1974) have put forth this argument. However, the logic of this point of view is faulty. It poses an either–or dichotomy—mental *or* neurological. People can comfortably speak of both a mental and a neurological illness if the mental and neurological characteristics are prominent enough to capture their attention. Neurologists of the future will probably be happy to restrict their practice to those neurological illnesses without severe and bizarre thought, which are feeling and behavior characteristics. Mental illness—with or without neurological illness—will still be handled by the psychiatrist.

The second way in which mental characteristics have been used to identify mental illness is more subtle. Often a patient complains of symptoms that, at first, point to a different type of illness. For example, a thirty-two-year-old woman was referred to a psychiatrist by her surgeon. Five months earlier, she underwent an abdominal operation. While the incision had healed nicely, it remained extraordinarily painful. It was even sensitive to the pressure of clothing. When the surgeon became convinced that the pain was not due to irritations of the healing process, he decided that psychiatric investigation was needed. A careful history revealed a pattern to the pain. It disturbed her sleep, causing her to awaken early in the morning. It bothered her during the day causing her appetite to diminish; food tasted bland and uninteresting. Sexual relations were out of the question because the contact would irritate the scar. She was so preoccupied by the problem that her usual wide-ranging activity schedule was severely constricted. The combination of symptoms pointed to an atypical depression — one of which even the patient was not aware. She was treated with antidepressant medication and psychotherapy and she made a rapid recovery. During the psychotherapy, she began to realize how vulnerable the operation had made her feel. She saw it as a punishment for angry wishes against her siblings, which she had harbored since childhood. Guilt had been mobilized, and with it was the irrational fear that she would be thrown out of her family. She had been convinced that she would never awaken from the anesthesia. Only after going beyond the most obvious complaint did the patient see how prominent the role of mental characteristics was.

The second bit of false reasoning set up by those who argue against the concept of mental illness may also be discussed. Are the illnesses real illnesses? The word *real* can have several meanings. It can mean genuine or bona fide; it can mean grounded in matter rather than imagination. The depressed patient did not have an illness grounded in the pathology of her incision. Her condition may even be conceived as being her imagination. However, this does not make it less genuine; it merely shifts the focus.

UNDESIRABILITY

The second criterion of illness — undesirability — can be considered after a cluster of prominent characteristics is focused upon and after they have been identified as being mental. Immediately, the psychiatrist must face the question, "undesirable to whom?" This is the problem of defining deviance — praiseworthy or dispraiseworthy behavior? — which was encountered in Chapter One. It is a problem of values rather than of scientific knowledge, although what is understood about the behavior in question will influence the way it is evaluated. The problem of determining whether a particular behavior cluster is desirable or undesirable can be illustrated with a graded series of situations.

First, the depressed person or the one who hears accusatory voices may be considered. These people spontaneously may seek relief from suffering. They evaluate the cluster of characteristics as undesirable. Their family, the psychiatrist, and society-at-large agree. There is a consensus — no dispute must be resolved.

Next, people with the cluster of characteristics known as mania may be evaluated. These people often do not feel the cluster is undesirable. They are elated, feel powerful, have more energy than usual, and have boundless optimism. However, they stand alone in their evaluation. Family, friends, and psychiatrists all disagree. There is a conflict here with the patient on one side and virtually everyone else on the other.

The area of personality disorders is the next step in this series. Usually people with these disorders do not feel that their behavior characteristics are undesirable. What society may call selfishness, they may call self-interest. Although a psychiatrist may see them as timid; they see themselves as cautious. Aggressiveness, to a professional, may be seen by them as defending one's rights. A psychiatrist's evaluation that their aloofness and social mistrustfulness is undesirable contrasts with their own evaluation that their lack of naiveté about the hypocrisy of others is desirable. Their cold-hearted lust for power may be decried, but they will respond that there is nothing wrong with ambition.

There are two differences between the situation with mania and that with personality disorders. First, while almost everyone would agree that the characteristics of the manic person are undesirable, there is not likely to be such unanimity with regard to personality characteristics. Second, the extent of the thinking and judgement disturbance in manic patients is so great that it is relatively easy for most observers to discount their ability to judge whether their behavior is desirable. The thinking of those with personality disorders is not so clearly irrational that their evaluations of their own behavior can be written off as resulting from a disturbed mind.

Last in the graded series are political or social dissenters. They do not feel that their characteristics are undesirable; indeed, they feel they are praiseworthy and so do many others who object to current social conditions. On the other hand, those who support the status quo are apt to evaluate the behavior as undesirable.

In this series, there is increasing disagreement about whether the behavior characteristics are undesirable. How can this issue be decided? Should a vote be taken? Should a professional be consulted, and if so, which professional? And how does the professional reach his or her conclusion? If the professional is a psychiatrist, does the process start by assessing that the person is sick and therefore in no condition to judge the desirability of his or her own behavior? That would involve circular reasoning, because in order to reach the first condition—illness, one must already have concluded that the behavior is undesirable.

Psychiatrists have no specific expertise in the realm of values. There is nothing in their training that gives them a special insight into the evaluation of desirability. Such evaluations are not scientific facts, they are opinions. Evaluations of desirability and undesirability rest largely on social policy.

With regard to the undesirability criterion of illness, then, three things can be concluded. (1) Some clusters of mental characteristics quite unequivocally fulfill this criterion; the target person and almost everyone else agree that the cluster is undesirable. However there are other conditions where there are differences of opinion. (2) While facts and understanding are important, ultimately the decision about whether the criterion is met is a matter of opinion and policy. (3) In the equivocal conditions, psychiatrists do not have specific training or expertise to decide whether the cluster is undesirable. The psychiatrist may describe and even explain the behavior, he or she may even be able to predict what the behavior is likely to lead to—the probable course. These are factual issues. But whether the cluster and its course is desirable or undesirable lies outside of the psychiatrist's area of expertise.

NATURAL AND RATIONAL COURSE

The third criterion of illness demands that the cluster of characteristics run a natural course with rationally understandable antecedents and outcomes. A disease theory is a deterministic theory. It does not say that all events in the universe are necessarily determined. However, those characteristics that are called illnesses are subject to the laws and regulations of cause and effect. They are determined, orderly, and rationally understandable.

Not all of the factors may be known in the chain of events. For example, all the processes leading to a particular type of cancer are not known, and certainly all the factors that are responsible for the course it takes are not known. In such cases, doctors and scientists operate out of conviction. They are convinced that orderly, rationally understandable sequences of natural events do occur and are yet to be discovered. Many clusters of mental characteristics fall into this category. While all the natural regulatory processes are not known, psychiatrists are convinced that they exist. There are causes, and the course and outcome of these conditions, while perhaps not predictable at present, are not arbitrary or matters of chance.

Friedson (1970, pp. 3ff.) has differentiated natural conditions from those where the explanations lie in the realm of the supernatural. Voodoo, witchcraft, possession, cures by exorcism, or miracles are supernatural; while many people believe in such phenomena, the prevailing view of illness is that illnesses are natural rather than supernatural processes. In this regard, it is of some interest that recently a Connecticut man charged with a crime pleaded not guilty, not by reason of insanity (illness), but by reason of demonic possession. He lost the case.

In former times, many of the behaviors that are now seen as mental illness were attributed to witchcraft and possession. It was only when more naturalistic explanations were discovered (or presumed to exist) that they were shifted into the illness category. Remnants of the possession theory are still observable in common language. When junior misbehaves, a parent may say, "I don't know what got into him today;" when a person is uneasy, he or she may say, "I'm not myself today."

In conditions with clear-cut, natural (usually biological) forces at work, there is little difficulty deciding that this third criterion of illness has been met. The depression, apathy, and confusion of hyperparathyroidism is directly related to an increase in the amount of calcium circulating in the bloodstream. With surgical removal of the parathyroid glands and a decrease in the serum calcium, the mental symptoms abate. Natural cause and effect is apparent. The cluster of undesirable mental characteristics meets the criterion of naturalism and rational understanding.

But what about the person who hears God or sees an angel during a phase of religious ecstasy? Is this natural or supernatural? Should the psychiatrist or the minister decide? Will each answer differently? How should the zealous religious leaders who are convinced that they have received divine inspiration to rid the world of what they see as immorality, sin, and anti-God political ideology be evaluated? Is this natural thought or spiritual revelation?

With regard to the naturalism criterion of illness, the same three conclusions can be reached as in the case of undesirability. (1) Some clusters of mental characteristics fulfill this criterion quite clearly; there is common agreement about causal processes. Other clusters are more equivocal; there may be legitimate differences of opinion. (2) In equivocal cases, whether a particular cluster is natural and rationally understandable is a matter of conviction, not fact. It is an opinion, however widely held—a policy. (3) Where there are differences of opinion, psychiatrists may not be able to demonstrate the natural orderly processes. They may have to decide out of conviction. Nothing in their training or expertise prepares them to decide the close calls or ambiguous cases.

BIOLOGICAL PROCESS

The fourth criterion of illness is that the cluster of characteristics under scrutiny should have a predominantly biological process as its focus. This condition is closely related to the third criterion—naturalism and orderly, understandable processes. However, whereas natural is contrasted with nonnatural (usually supernatural), biological as used here is usually contrasted with psychological. The question to be confronted here is whether psychological processes are or are not biological.

Earlier in this chapter, the faulty dichotomy of mental versus neurological or mental versus physical was discussed. The position was taken that certain clusters of mental characteristics could require the focus on important bodily processes as well—

mental and biological. Clearly, the mental characteristics of hyperparathyroidism require a biological focus. Drug-induced hallucinations, paranoia, and excitement and the orientation and memory disturbances of an individual whose brain is being crowded and compressed by a blood clot are further examples of the fallacy of the either–or approach.

There are several mental conditions in which the evidence of strong biological underpinnings, while not conclusive, is at least suggestive. In some of these, the medications employed to treat the conditions have given valuable clues about the neurochemical processes regulating the mental characteristics. Schizophrenia and the major affective disorders (mania and severe depression) are examples. In addition to the chemical approach, family studies suggest that several conditions (clusters of mental characteristics) may be transmitted genetically. Schizotypal individuals, although not actually psychotic, are marked by social isolation, awkward and peculiar use of language, and a tendency to have mystical or magical feelings. There is some evidence that people with this cluster of mental characteristics (which is termed a personality disorder [DSM III]) may be related genetically to people with schizophrenia (Kety et al., 1968). It may be that these individuals have the same type of biological processes but with lesser intensity. Likewise, cyclothymic individuals whose moods alternate between moderate elation and high spirit on the one hand and mild depression, listlessness, and discouragement on the other seem to be related genetically to people with the major affective disorders (Akiskal, 1981). Even antisocial personality disorder—that vexing category with which Doctors Overholser and Duval grappled—may have some genetic (and thus biological) basis, although the evidence is still very slim (Heston, 1966; Cloninger et al., 1975).

But even if some mental conditions are also biological, are all of them? Can there be some clusters of mental characteristics that are not biological at all? For example, what about learned patterns of behavior for which no basis in anatomy, chemistry, physics, or genetics can be demonstrated? What about undesirable ideas and emotions, and the behavior that may proceed from them? Is it possible to have a deviant mind without having a deviant brain?

There is no answer to that question and probably there never will be. This is the entrance into the realm of philosophy that considers the relationship between mental and physical processes. Of the many ways philosophers have conceptualized the relationship between mind and body (Gotschalk, 1968, pp. 220ff.; Popper and Eccles, 1977, Part I), two shall be considered here; interactionism and identity. Although they are exceedingly complex conceptualizations, they are presented here in grossly oversimplified fashion. For the purpose of carrying forth the discussion, it is sufficient to contrast them.

The interactionist view (Popper and Eccles, 1977) maintains there are two separate realms — mental, which is not material or localizable in space, and physical. In this view, mental and physical are opposites — either one or the other, but not both. Sometimes, however, they interact. Much of the time, they pursue relatively independent courses. Indeed, the mental realm may not even be subject to the regulation of cause and effect; it is a different type of thing from the physical realm. In this view, while interaction might give some clusters of mental characteristics a significant biological focus, there could be other mental clusters pursuing their own course without significant biological characteristics. One could indeed have a deviant mind without having a deviant brain.

The identity view (Feigl, 1967) does not refer to two separate realms. In fact, as Langer (1967, pp. 21ff.) explains, mental activity should not be described by nouns, such as *realm* or *mind.* Even such nouns as *thought* or *feeling* are misleading because they seem to refer to things. (However, for linguistic convenience, the use of these terms will be continued.) Thinking and feeling are activities; they are functions of the organisms, much in the same way that pumping is a function of the heart. Langer refers to these activities as phases while Gotschalk (1968, pp. 231ff.) calls them qualities. The *thing* is the brain and it can exist in two phases — aware and unaware. Langer analogizes mental activity to the redness in red hot iron. When the iron is heated hot enough, it is in the red phase; when it cools, it is not in the red phase.

This view does not pose two opposite things or realms. There is only one thing — a brain. In the identity view, both mental *or* biological and mental *and* biological are poor formulations; mental *is* biological. Although there can be biological without mental (the iron without red), there can be no mental without biological (the red without iron). From this point of view, it is not possible to have deviant mental characteristics without a deviant brain.

These are two philosophical points of view; they are not facts but conceptualizations. Nothing in the training of psychiatrists prepares them to choose one or the other theory. It becomes a matter of opinion, not expertise.

Many writers claim that only those clusters of mental characteristics that obviously are based biologically are illnesses; the nonbiological clusters are problems of living. These writers unwittingly proceed from an interactionist point of view. That is their privilege, of course, but their position represents an opinion, and not even an expert opinion, for it is equally possible to adopt the identity viewpoint and declare that all mental characteristics are biological.

Even the identity theorist might wish to distinguish between biological and psychological on the basis of the phenomenon of learning. One might take the position that the brain made deviant by infection or trauma represents a biological process while the brain made deviant by message inputs (learning) is not a biological process. Others, however, might object to this differentiation. When other organs are made deviant by message inputs, there is no difficulty in attributing a biological process and illness. For example, the heart attack triggered by bad news, the high blood pressure maintained by chronic stress, and the many diseases resulting in great measure from culturally derived patterns of living are not less biological because the organs become deviant due to message inputs.

With regard to the biological criterion of illness, then, three things may be concluded. (1) Some clusters of mental characteristics quite unequivocally fulfill this criterion; almost everyone agrees they have a biological base. However, there are other conditions where there are differences of opinion. (2) While facts and understanding are important, ultimately the decision about whether the criterion is met is a matter of opinion and policy. (3) In the equivocal conditions, psychiatrists do not have specific training or expertise to decide whether the cluster is biological.

INDIVIDUAL FOCUS

The fifth criterion of illness is that the cluster of characteristics must have a predominately individual rather than a social focus. Since the mental characteristics most often are played out on the social stage and the behavior under scrutiny often is triggered by events in the individual's surroundings, should the focus be on the processes within the individual or those between the individual and the people with whom he or she interacts (social)? To simplify this discussion, the identity viewpoint that considers all mental processes within the individual to be biological should be assumed.

Once again, a graded series may be examined. In the case of mental confusion of a person with a brain tumor, it can be agreed reasonably that the focus of the characteristics lies with the individual. This individual would be confused in any social setting.

Next schizophrenia will be examined. Scheff (1966) has taken the position that many of the characteristics of the cluster called schizophrenia do not so much represent a state or trait of the individual; much of the cluster is a role forced on him or her by a society that has branded the person with such a stigmatizing label. While such a labelling theory has been amply rebutted (Wing, 1978, Chapters 4 and 5), and while there is evidence pointing to an individual focus in schizophrenia, there is no question that the behavior also is shaped by the social surroundings.

In the area of anxiety disorders, the focus of the problem may be even more equivocal. For example, agoraphobia—the intense fright at the prospect of leaving the house—may be treatable by medication, by behavioral psychotherapy, or by family therapy. While the response to medication of some people with agoraphobia suggests that the problem is biological, the response to alterations in the family relationships suggests it may be social.

Personality disorders can pose particular difficulties of focus. As Frances (1980) has pointed out, when trying to assess the personality of someone, a psychiatrist must attempt to differentiate between trait and role. A black adolescent charged with rape may be so scared because of his situation and so intimidated by the older, white examining psychiatrist that he appears timid, hesitant, passive, and submissive. In his more usual setting, he may be active, bossy, and ready to take risks. Are the characteristics predominately rooted in the young man or in the social setting — trait or role? And even more longer-lasting characteristics, traits such as ambition, dominance, assertiveness, can also be seen as roles defined by a person's place in society — social class, education level, etc.

This graded series, then, illustrates that social factors may play a minimal role in the cluster of characteristics under scrutiny or may be of greater and greater importance. Where the line is drawn or where the balance has tilted so far toward the social that illness can no longer be spoken of is strictly a matter of opinion. There are no factual guidelines; there is no expertise in the grey area.

Thus, when the fourth criterion of illness is applied–individual rather than social focus — the same three familiar conclusions are made. (1) Some clusters of mental characteristics clearly fulfill the individual criterion. Other clusters, however, are more ambiguous. (2) In many cases, whether a cluster of mental characteristics is individual rests on opinion and conviction. It is a policy decision, depending on how much weight is given to the social factors. (3) Where there are differences of opinion, once the relevant facts are laid out, the psychiatrist has no special training that enables him or her to resolve the issue; there is no expertise in deciding the close calls.

LACK OF CONTROL

The sixth criterion of illness is that the cluster of characteristics be beyond the control of the individual; he or she cannot change the characteristics by willpower. As Wing (1978, pp. 44ff.) put it, there is a continuum of mental reactions; some are mild, some are severe. There is a point, however, where there is an "inability to stop the syndrome by *deliberately* turning the attention to something else" (italics added). Beyond this point lies illness.

Like the criteria of naturalism and biology, this condition rests on the issue of determinism — cause and effect. Strict determinists would say that all human activity (including thought, feeling, and behavior) proceeds *inevitably*, governed by inescapable natural laws. There is no such thing as choice, willpower, control of the individual, or deliberately doing anything. People are passive reactors; behavior is compelled.

An alternate position has been termed *libertarianism* by Broad (1952)*. This viewpoint is a type of soft determinism, which acknowledges that an individual's actions are partly determined by what has gone before, who the person is, and what information he or she receives from the surroundings. However, at some point this casual chain is interrupted and the person consciously and willfully chooses his/her behavioral actions. Although all the determinants may be considered, the individual is not locked into any one possibility. He or she can exercise free will. People are active deciders; they control their behavior. However, there are certain circumstances over which the person has no control; in a sense, the determinants are too strong and override the ability to make a free choice. This situation will be referred to as the *crippling of the choosing mechanism*. When the choosing mechanism is crippled, when the person is not in control of his or her actions, behavior is compelled and the deterministic requirement is met. When this happens, illness may occur. When the choosing mechanism is intact, poor choices may occur but this is not illness.

Some, such as Szasz (1961), Hampshire (1965), and Schafer (1978) take the view that virtually all mental characteristics are chosen and the feeling of inevitable forces is an illusion. Most people take a libertarian view that humans usually are able to consider and weigh what has gone before and then make a free choice; at times, however, a person may be sick and his/her choosing mechanism is crippled. Still others (Mandler and Kessen, 1974) hold the view that all thought, feeling, and behavior is regulated by cause and effect; choice is an illusion. Which position each individual adopts is a matter of conviction. There is no fact or expertise in this area. And yet, only if the libertarian stance is adopted is there even hope to distinguish between mental illness and nonillness.

Even if, out of conviction and belief, the libertarian view is

---

*While Broad maintains that the libertarian position is not possible (a view not held by the author), it is the viewpoint held by most people and the framework in which most *sick or* _____? questions are asked.

adopted, there may be problems deciding whether any particular behavior was freely chosen or inevitably and uncontrollably determined. Consider the example of Mrs. Litton, who had come for treatment because she was unable to feel successful at her job or to enjoy dating. While she was a very self-centered woman, her self-esteem was fragile and she was prone to severe feelings of disappointment when she was not praised or helped by those she viewed more powerful than herself.

When she was nineteen, she had married a bright, charismatic person who had a meteoric rise in industry. She lived in his shadow and basked in his glory. Ultimately he divorced her and left her with two children. However, she still placed him on a pedestal and longed for his return.

People such as Mrs. Litton, who overidealize their spouses and cannot let them go even when they are unequivocally told the relationship has ended, may harbor considerable rage of which they are unaware. On occasion, this rage may suddenly peak and an ordinarily unaggressive person may commit violence (Bursten, 1981).

One day, Mrs. Litton was extremely frustrated. She again had called her husband to suggest that they get together for a weekend to talk things over. He had declined gently but firmly. Later that day, she was combing her hair before a mirror when she gradually was overcome by an urge to murder her husband. She described the feeling as "eerie." She kept looking in the mirror to see if it were really she who was having these thoughts—it was so unlike her to think of violence and to cast her husband in a negative light. The idea became a preoccupation, and she literally shook her head in an attempt to get rid of it. The urge became stronger and stronger; she felt possessed. Fortunately a telephone call from a friend shook her out of the trance. The patient could not explain her feeling; she tended to disown it. But she was convinced that it was so powerful that she might have killed her husband were it not for the interruption. And the whole experience left her terribly frightened.

Could Mrs. Litton choose to control herself and not become violent? Although she did not act on her impulse, this may not have been because of her decision. It may have been a result of the telephone call that interrupted the impulsive thoughts. This was no choice at all. But what if there had not been an interruption? What if she had killed her husband? Would psychiatrists say the trance or the impulse crippled her choosing mechanism and she went out of control? Or would they say that she became so angry that she chose to kill him? How can the answer possibly be established?

Psychiatrists are not trained to detect whether a person could or could not have chosen to act differently from the way he or she actually acted. They study the natural course of mental illness, the influence of past and present experience on behavior, the biological underpinnings, etc. All these are factual matters based on whatever knowledge the profession has accumulated about cause and effect. Professional expertise lies in the deterministic mode of formulation. This does not mean that all psychiatrists are determinists; it does mean, however, that psychiatry can describe many things about human beings, but the ability to choose is not included in this description. There are no reliable guidelines to determine which person can choose and which person cannot. According to Robitscher (1968), "A psychiatrist . . . can give details of previous mental troubles, trace the course of a developing illness, demonstrate the ego deficiencies—all of which may indicate a defendant may have found an impulse more irresistable than might a man with a stronger ego. But the point at which the impulse crosses the borderline from resistability to irresistability is not a determination for the psychiatrist; it is only able to be made in the abstract by a meta-physician and in the concrete by a judge and jury."

Even this should be analyzed further because *ego deficiencies* and *stronger ego* do not add any clarity. There are some who suggest that people with strong egos can control themselves and can exercise freedom of choice while those with weak egos are determined much more strictly. But how is ego strength measured? It usually is measured in terms of the very behavior used to explain it. If a person's actions suggest that he or she has self-control, he or she has a strong ego; if the person acts impulsively, usually psychiatrists say he or she has a weaker ego.

In 1954, the Group of the Advancement of Psychiatry (GAP,

1954) suggested that "ego impairment would appear to be a direct measure of responsibility." Nevertheless, the authors maintain that it is not possible to construct a measure of ego impairment. Therefore, they concluded that the concept of ego impairment does not enable psychiatrists to assign responsibility.

With regard to the absence of control and willpower criterion of illness, once again the same conclusions are reached. (1) The question arises only if a libertarian viewpoint is adopted. For the strict determinists, the criterion is always met. For those who feel all behavior is chosen, the criterion is never met. Within the libertarian framework, some clusters of mental characteristics impress virtually everyone as being compelled. Usually these are the bizarre characteristics, out of character, and with obvious biological underpinnings. Other clusters, however, are more ambiguous. (2) Whether a libertarian position is adopted is a matter of policy, not fact. Within the libertarian framework, whether the ambiguous case is viewed as compelled or chosen rests on opinion, not fact. (3) Psychiatrists cast behavior in the deterministic framework of science. They do not have special expertise that allows them to judge whether a libertarian framework might be applicable. And even when they adopt a libertarian position, their expertise does not help them decide whether an equivocal cluster of mental characteristics was compelled or chosen.

Thus, it is possible to define a cluster of mental characteristics. In some clear-cut cases, there is general agreement that the other five criteria—undesirability, naturalness and rational understandability, biology, individual focus, and absence of control and willpower—have been met. In these situations, it is justifiable to use the term *mental illness.* However, in many ambiguous situations, those four criteria may be evaluated differently by different people. Facts help only up to a point; ultimately the criteria rest on opinion and policy. Training does not provide psychiatrists with relevant expertise. They are not in a better position to decide whether the ambiguous clusters meet these five criteria.

In other words, in equivocal cases, the decision to call a cluster of mental characteristics mental illness is a matter of policy. The fiasco perpetrated by Doctors Overholser and Duval may not have been such a fiasco after all. It may have been a reasonable reaction to having been asked impossible questions by a society that needed to have answers even if they were not based on fact. For the present, then, society must remain with the disturbing conclusion that in many of the crucial decision-making situations, there is no scientific or factual way of saying whether a particular person has mental illness. It is a matter of policy.

CHAPTER THREE

PRODUCT

In the previous chapter, the conclusion was made that some clusters of mental characteristics so clearly fit the criteria of illness that most psychiatrists agree to categorize them as mental illness. Other clusters are ambiguous, and opinion about whether the illness criteria are satisfied will be divided sharply. In the equivocal cases, expertise fails because these are issues of policy rather than of scientific fact. But the problem does not stop there. The *Durham* standard is *product of mental illness*. Just what is meant by *product?* As the court in *Carter v United States* (1957) said, the fact that a person has a mental disease does not necessarily mean that every action he or she engages in results from that mental illness; "there must be a relationship between the disease and the act, and that relationship, whatever it may be in degree, must be . . . decisive, determinative, causal . . . "

What does a "decisive, determinative, causal" relationship imply? At the very least, it suggests that a mentally ill person's actions (the products) may be separate in some way from the illness, or that there may be decisive factors in addition to the illness that prompted the action. The word *product* becomes a bit more complex. In this chapter, a closer look will be taken at the concept of *product* and there will be a discussion of the problems encountered when psychiatrists attempt to use this concept in the practical, decision-making situations described in Chapter One.

Despite what was concluded in the previous chapter, for the purposes of the discussion of *product* the reader should assume there is no difficulty in identifying a cluster of mental characteristics as illness. Having thus identified a particular person as mentally ill, a series of questions that relate to the *product* concept can be generated.

1. Is the particular behavior under scrutiny a product of the illness or a feature of it?
2. Can an action be caused by ideas?
3. Can a person be partly mentally ill and partly well?
4. If a person can be partly mentally ill and partly well, how is a specific behavior between the sick and healthy parts allocated?
5. How should a psychiatrist distinguish between behavior that is a direct product of illness and that which is in reaction to the illness?

Here, then, are a few of the issues that are contained in the concept *product*. While some of them may be of greater interest to philosophers, most of them have relevance to the clinical and legal situations that psychiatrists are likely to encounter.

PRODUCT OR FEATURE OF ILLNESS?

Is the particular behavior under scrutiny a product of the mental illness or a feature of it? If the behavior is a product of the illness, a causal chain results: X causes Y. A causal chain requires at least two identifiable elements. The first is the cause and the second is the effect or product.

Consider the woman who sits in a psychiatrist's office and rubs her hands back and forth on the arms of the chair. She then thumps the table hard with her knuckles. When she becomes psychotic, things do not seem real to her. She is not certain where she ends and the outside world begins. She needs to feel the firmness of the chair and the hardness of the table to help her define the boundary between self and nonself. Is her behavior caused by her mental illness or is it part of it? Is this a product or feature of mental illness? Remember, mental characteristics have been defined as thought, feelings, *and* behavior.

Another example is the man who is apathetic, easily startled, subject to irritable outbursts and nightmares. The behavior under scrutiny is his failure to go to work. The problem started when a scaffold on which he was standing at the factory suddenly collapsed and he narrowly escaped death. Is the act of staying home a separate element caused by the posttraumatic stress disorder or is it a feature of it?

In the immediate aftermath of *Durham*, several psychiatrists (e.g. Wertham, 1955; Roche, 1955, 1956) took the position that the mental illness and the act under scrutiny were not two different elements but were one. As Roche (1955) said, "Mental illness does not cause one to commit a crime nor does mental illness produce a crime. Behavior and mental illness are inseparable—one and the same thing."

In terms of the issues with which this book is concerned, the *one element or two?* question is a pseudoproblem. Whether the behavior under scrutiny is viewed as a product or a feature of the mental illness makes no practical difference. Given a person with a mental illness, the only crucial question is whether the behavior under scrutiny was inevitable or whether it was chosen.

In terms of one element, the behavior is a feature of the mental illness. By definition, it is inevitable because sickness is determined, not chosen. In terms of two elements, the behavior is deemed to be the product of the illness. The illness caused the behavior in a "decisive, determinative" manner. It was still inevitable.

On the other side of the coin, in terms of one element it may be concluded that, despite the mental illness, this particular behavior is not a sign or feature of it. The individual may have been sick, but he or she chose his or her behavior. With regard to the activity under scrutiny, the label *sick* will be rejected and instead it will be referred to as *sinful, unwise,* etc. In terms of two elements, although the person is mentally ill, this particular behavior is not a product of it.

Another way of pointing up this issue as a pseudoproblem is to view it in terms of a *but for* analysis. In many areas of the law, the question of a causal connection is phrased *But for the occurrence of X, would Y have occurred?* When considering *But for occurrence of mental illness, the behavior under scrutiny would not have occurred,* it does not matter whether the behavior is viewed as an effect of the illness or as a feature of it.

For the sake of convenience, the word *product,* which can be interpreted to mean consequence, effect (causal relationship between two elements) or feature, sign of illness (one element) will continue to be used. The important point to bear in mind is the crucial question of inevitability. Given the mental illness, was the individual compelled to behave the way he or she did? Impairment in deciding, choosing, or exercising free will is the critical issue. Given mental illness, *product of mental illness* implies that the behavior in question resulted from a crippled choosing mechanism.

CAUSES OR REASONS?

Can an action be caused by ideas? There are some (Ryle, 1949; Melden, 1961; Hampshire, 1965; Schafer, 1978) who insist that ideas cannot cause anything. These writers distinguish between causes on the one hand and reasons and contexts on the other. A cause has the inevitability of determinism. A reason or context does not inevitably lead to action. It is considered, but then the person makes his or her own free decision—chooses what action to take. This is a libertarian view. Since the causal chain between ideas and action was interrupted by an independent decision that inevitably was not tied to the ideas, these ideas are reasons or explanations of the action—they are the context in which the action was taken—but they are not causes. The behavior is not inevitably tied to the ideas; despite the individual's thoughts and grasp of the situation, he or she could have chosen to act differently.

It is common for people to refer to their thoughts in causal terms. "I stopped the car *because* I saw the red light and I knew what that meant." However, according to the libertarian view, given the same perceptions and understanding, "I could have run the light. I chose to stop." The ideas did not cause the action; there was no inevitability. Indeed, this is the basis for morality; "If I had run the light, I would have been bad."

Schafer (1978, pp. 73ff.) has maintained that when humans feel they have lost the ability to choose (e.g. when ideas are so overwhelming that they compel action), they are merely under an illusion. It is a person's way of disclaiming personal responsibility for actions about which he or she is ashamed or guilty. As previously noted, Schafer belongs to the philosophical group that says all behavior is chosen; ideas may provide a context for the choice, but they cause no behavior. If this view is adopted, all *product* questions vanish because the choosing mechanism is never crippled. Even if the individual's ideas are bizarre and they fit the criteria of mental illness, the action is neither a feature of the illness nor is it caused by the ideas, because all actions are freely chosen.

On the other hand, since all behavior occurs in a mental context, it is possible to view every action as caused by ideas. Every act is determined; there is no choice. In this case, all undesirable acts would be seen as *products of mental illness*. Once again, the *sick or* _____? questions would vanish.

While either of these absolutist positions might be comfortable for professional psychiatrists, society holds to a middle road. All the *sick or* _____? questions assume that when the constellation of ideas (and feelings) meet the criteria of illness, these ideas have the possibility of causing the action if the choosing mechanism is crippled, or not causing the action if the person is capable of making a free decision. If the ideas caused the action, the person is sick; if the ideas merely provided the context but the individual made a choice, he or she is not sick but sinful, unwise, etc. Once again, psychiatrists are asked to step into the murky realm of questions about inevitability—a realm in which they have no training or expertise.

PARTIAL MENTAL ILLNESS

Can a person be partly mentally ill and partly well? Is there such a condition as partial insanity, or is it more nearly accurate to consider a person either mentally ill or not? This question is of considerable importance because the significance of *product* will vary according to the answer. If the whole person is considered to be mentally ill, all his or her actions are *products of mental illness*. However, in the case of partial illness, the problem arises of whether the behavior in question proceeded from the sick aspect or the healthy aspect. Partial mental illness can be diagrammed as shown in Figure 1.

One could argue that an action is performed by a person as an integrated whole and not by part of a person (e.g. Schafer, 1978).

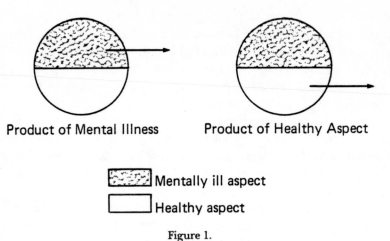

Product of Mental Illness   Product of Healthy Aspect

Mentally ill aspect

Healthy aspect

Figure 1.

There is a large body of psychoanalytic data demonstrating that even if the mind is compartmentalized in theory, each part influences the functioning of every other part.

However, common sense contradicts this concept. There can be sick and healthy aspects of mental functioning within the same individual. For example, an anxious young man seeks help because he senses something strange is happening; he cannot concentrate, he hears voices, and things often look unreal to him. He is given medicine to take three times a day. He agrees, and he has understood and will follow directions. This is the healthy aspect—the aspect in which reality can be grasped. Indeed, the very fact that he realizes something is wrong suggests that certain mental functions remain intact. This is not to suggest that there is a mind with different parts, some sick and some healthy, as if the mind had geographical properties. The mind can be pictured in that fashion only metaphorically, as Freud (1923) did; indeed, Figure 1 is a metaphor; it is to be used as a tool of communication rather than a statement of reality.

This view of mental functioning has been reflected in the law. The court in *State u Jones* (1871) determined that "in most of the cases which come before the courts, where it is sufficiently apparent that disease has attacked the mind in some form and to some extent, it has not thus wholly obliterated the will, the conscience, and the mental power, but has left its victim still in possession of some degree of ability in some or all of these qualities ... the term, partial insanity, has been applied to such cases. ... "

In any individual, some mental functions may be intact and others may be compromised. As knowledge of the neurological underpinnings of mental functions increases, relatively specific areas of the brain may be found to be involved in certain mental illnesses. This does not mean that mental functions subserved by other areas are unaffected; severe dysfunction in one sphere must influence a person's entire functioning. What it does suggest, however, is that even if one set of mental functions is disturbed seriously, other mental functions may not be disturbed so severely that they meet the criteria of illness set forth in Chapter Two.

Traditionally, there are three areas of mental functioning that have been examined when society has turned to psychiatrists for help in decision making: cognition, emotion, and impulsivity. The cognitive area deals with the information an individual has when the action is contemplated and executed. Behavior is the motion of an individual in a context and the person's understanding or appraisal of that context reflects his or her cognition. Cognitive functioning is concerned with ideas; it comprises the processing of information from the social surround.

Information processing may be faulty in several areas. Delusions (false beliefs), hallucinations, defects in memory, problems in orientation (appreciation of time, place, person and situation), inability to concentrate or to calculate, and difficulty in employing syllogistic reasoning or in slowing down one's racing thoughts are some of the problems of cognition.

A man observed that his landlord failed to collect the rent at the usual time. He became suspicious and sought the landlord. He found him conversing in a low tone to a seedy-looking character and he suddenly realized that a drug transaction was taking place. As he left the scene, it occurred to him that the landlord may have seen him and would want to kill him to keep him from talking. There was nothing to do but quickly to pack his belongings and to flee the city. As he drove off, he noticed that he had to stop at every red light. He thought the landlord must have had cohorts who were trying to hinder his flight. He drove through several states, pausing only to get gas. But the drug conspirators had spread the word and he could tell by the way the gas station attendants were looking at him that they were telephoning his whereabouts back to the headquarters of the drug ring. Finally, after driving all night, he arrived in a large city on a Saturday morning. He went straight to police headquarters, but they did not seem to take his story seriously. He did not know what to do, but somehow he had to let the government know. Since narcotics traffic is a federal offense, he went to a federal building, but it was closed. In desperation, he crashed his car into the glass doors of the building, knowing that in this way he would at least get to talk with federal officials.

This man misunderstood his situation. He could not process information received from the environment in a realistic manner. While he knew he was crashing into a federal building, the information he relied on to frame the context of the behavior was faulty. His mental illness lay in the cognitive sphere. Now, suppose the police had given him the correct information. While he would have had the realistic information, he would not have believed it. He would still have acted on the basis of his belief in the faulty information. Thus, cognition requires more than having been provided with the correct context; it requires belief.

Most psychiatrists would agree that the complex of mental characteristics exhibited by this man met the criteria of illness set forth in Chapter Two. The disturbances were in the cognitive area. The cues he received from his surroundings were processed in a faulty manner. However, not all of his cognitive functioning was delusional. He recognized red lights for what they were. He was able to drive safely and purposefully through several states. He reasoned quite correctly that crashing into the doors of a federal building would gain him the attention of the authorities. While some of his cognition was dysfunctional, some was quite functional—he was partly sick and partly well. However, even some of his rational thinking was influenced by delusions. While he was able to process correctly the many cues necessary to locate the federal building, to aim the car, to anticipate some of the consequences, etc., his understanding of the context of the behavior was sick. Given this faulty information processing system, what can be said about his ability to choose his actions? Was the crash determined, in a causal sense, by this information? Could this man have chosen not to act this way? Assuming that ideas can in some circumstances cause behavior, there is still no accurate way of determining whether this individual's ideas so affected his ability to make choices such that his choosing mechanism was crippled or overridden.

The second area of mental functioning is that of the emotions. While behavior can be termed healthy when it occurs in the context of a variety of emotions, there are certain situations in which the emotional coloring is called an illness. The depression and despair of a suicidal patient is a case in point. The eruptive rage of certain violent men (Bursten, 1981) in some cases might be seen as unhealthy, as is the euphoria of a manic patient and the irritability of the depressed person. Guilt is sometimes so compelling that it leads to actions that cause downfall (Freud, 1915).

Although many schizophrenic people display emotions so at variance with their thoughts that they may be judged as peculiar, the emotions of most other people deviate from the normal range not in quality but in intensity. Put very simply, how strong must an emotion be in order to conclude that it overpowered the choosing mechanism?

The third area of mental functioning which commands attention is that of impulsivity. The term *urge* is preferred to *impulse* because it refers to the initiation of an action whether it is relatively spontaneous or subsequent to a long period of brooding or planning.

People tend to think that the urge to action is entirely dependent on cognitive and emotional processes. If one type of information is processed, an action may be prompted; other information may lead to delay and provide time for reflection. If emotions are strong enough, action is taken; less strong emotions allow for temporary deference of action.

However, there are some indications that, in addition to cognitive and emotional input into the initiation of action, there may be urge mechanisms that give an individual generally a higher or lower readiness to action. Some people are able to control their anger, some have the urge to act. Often, alcohol inhibits the control mechanisms. Certain subtle brain dysfunctions can result in disinhibitions (Monroe, 1978) and automatic behavior even when there is no cognitive deficit (Feldman, 1981).

Kornhuber (1974) has described "readiness potentials," which are characteristic patterns of electrical activity recorded from the brain just prior to an action. Eccles (Popper and Eccles, 1977, p. 285) suggests that this electrical activity may represent the brain in a "Go now!" state. For example, eating is subject to start and stop mechanisms that are not dependent entirely on context and emotion (Pribram, 1971, pp. 187ff). If, indeed, there are "start and stop switches" in the brain, it is not at all impossible that they could be set at faster or slower levels by biological development, injury, or input from previous experience as well as by present cognition or emotion.

One might consider kleptomania as a specific deficit in the urge mechanism. A person with this condition might be able to restrain most actions. However, this individual may steal a cheap item from a store despite the fact that he or she could well afford to pay for it and does not really need it. There is no unreality in the information, and while the emotion may be one of mounting excitement, the shoplifter is usually left saying, "I don't know why I did it; I just could not control the urge." Many sex offenders are subject to similar kinds of impulsivity. Manic people may have more generalized difficulty with restraint. They are frequently quick to convert thought into action. Their information processing and emotionality are also faulty, but beyond that, much of their activity is so driven and seems so peremptory that it is not difficult to infer a broad deficit in the functioning of the urge mechanisms.

Once again, the difference between normal urge mechanisms and urge settings that are too fast is one of degree rather than of quality. There is no scientific way to determine the point of which the urge mechanisms have been set so high that the ability to choose is compromised.

When these three broad areas of mental functioning are considered, some differences are apparent. While the emotion and urge functions are put to the test of illness with regard to their intensity, the cognitive functions are put to the test of illness by their quality. With regard to any particular action, the question must be asked whether the emotion or urge was so strong that it impaired the actor's ability to choose. However, in the realm of cognition, the question that must be asked is if the information processing was so different from the way people generally process information that the ability to choose was impaired.

This difference between urge and emotion on the one hand and cognition on the other has practical consequences. In deciding whether an action was the *product of mental illness*, the particular mental characteristics that are disturbed must be examined. A person with very strong rage or impulse is expected to control him or herself. After all, everyone has experienced anger or urge to action and have behaved. The public is less ready to accept behavior resulting from disturbances in these spheres as *products of mental illness*. However, the person with delusions, the person who does not know where he or she is or who cannot speak an intelligible sentence readily can be seen as different from the norm of society. Therefore, the behavior evoked by the disturbance in cognition is accepted more readily as a *product of mental illness*. However, there is no scientific or logical reason to conclude that cognitive impairments should be treated as mental illness while intense emotional and urge functions should not. This distinction rests on common sense — it seems right and fair to many people. It is a matter of policy.

ALLOCATION OF BEHAVIOR

If a person can be partly mentally ill and partly well, how is a specific behavior allocated between the sick and the healthy parts? For the purpose of this discussion, the reader should assume the libertarian philosophical position outlined earlier in this chapter. The word *influence* will be used to refer to the effect of either sick or healthy thoughts, feelings, and urges on behavior. If the behavior was influenced by the healthy functions, it was chosen. Healthy functions can provide the context in which a decision is made, but the choosing mechanism is not impaired by the context. If the behavior was influenced by the sick part, it was caused in a deterministic sense because impairment of the choosing mechanism and cause and effect are criteria by which sick clusters of mental characteristics have been defined.

The present problem has two stages. First, a particular behavior must be examined to see if it was influenced by the sick part or the healthy part. This is the initial allocation. However, often the situation is not either–or. The behavior in question reasonably may be allocated to both sick and well functions. Then, the second stage, *allocation of product,* must be presented to decide whether the influence of the sick or the healthy part predominated.

Looking at the first stage of allocation, how can a specific behavior be attached to a particular sick or well cluster of mental functions? The first test of this stage is that of reasonableness. If the action makes sense in terms of the ideas, it was caused by the idea (sick part) or chosen in the context of the idea (healthy part). For example, one day a quiet and seclusive young man unaccountably went to the apartment of a neighbor whom he did not know. When the woman answered the bell, he stabbed her to death. Holding the bloody knife aloft as a banner, he ran into the street and shouted triumphantly. He was surprised when he was apprehended and treated as a criminal instead of a hero. He explained that he was prompted to do the act by his conviction that women are the embodiment of all evil in the world and that God had informed him it was his role to purge the world of this evil. Killing even one woman—any woman—would be a symbolic act signifying man's triumph over evil. Given such a delusion (sick part), the action makes sense and the behavior can be attributed to that particular cluster of mental characteristics. One does not have to be a psychiatrist to test reasonableness; it is not a matter of expertise. There is a second test of this stage that is applied when behavior is allocated to the sick part. Usually, psychiatrists examine the cluster of mental characteristics in question and see if they fit a diagnostic category. The hero, for example, heard voices, believed that he was controlled by mysterious influences, and had other characteristics of paranoid schizophrenia. It is known that a fair number of people with paranoid schizophrenia commit offenses such as stabbing. Most people with paranoid schizophrenia are not violent, but violence is not unusual. Using this quasi-statistical standard, it could be said that the behavior was at least consistent with the diagnosis.

This second test becomes even more important when the sick

cluster of mental characteristics is not ideas (cognition). The emotional irresistibility of some people with clinical depression or the high urge setting of people with mania may trigger actions that are difficult to explain in terms of reasonable relation to ideas. Psychiatrists feel more at ease allocating specific behaviors to the sick part if their experience has taught them that such behavior is consistent with the diagnosis.

When it comes to allocating behavior to sick mental functions, then, psychiatrists do have some expertise. They have a body of knowledge, based on experience, which indicates that certain behaviors are consistent with certain other clusters of mental characteristics to which a diagnostic label is given.

In the example of the "hero," suppose the circumstances were different. Suppose that in addition to his instructions to purge the world of evil women, he actually knew this woman. Suppose that she owed him money and refused to pay. He became angry and bitter. He had told a friend that he would "get her." Now, the stabbing could be reasonably understood in terms of the healthy functions as well. While most people would have controlled their resentment, he chose to get his revenge in a manner that logically was related to his cognitions. In this situation, then, the test of reasonableness allowed the allocation of the behavior to the healthy part. Of course, the second test (consistency with the diagnosis) cannot be applied because there probably was no diagnosis, or if there was a well diagnosis, stabbing would never be consistent with it.

When behavior is allocated to the healthy functions, psychiatrists may be helpful because they know how to find information in interviews, but the test of reasonableness needs no expertise. Given the explanation of the situation, psychiatrists and non-psychiatrists alike may allocate to the healthy part.

If the hero's behavior can be allocated both to the sick part and the healthy part, the question of how to apportion the influence of each part on the choosing mechanism arises. This is the second stage of allocation. Was the choosing mechanism overridden; was the behavior a *product of mental illness?* Or was the sick part so insignificant in proportion to the healthy part that the man was able to choose to commit the offense?

There is no expertise that can help in apportioning the influences of the sick and healthy functions on behavior. Nothing in their training enables psychiatrists to ascertain how much influence each function has, or just at what point the choosing mechanism is so crippled that it was rendered ineffective. The point at which a certain behavior becomes inevitable is not a scientific issue. Nonetheless, this weighing of allocations between sick and well and coming up with a single answer must be done. The *sick or* _____*?* questions described in Chapter One cannot be answered by saying, "The patient is partly sick and partly sinful, unwise, etc." Such a conclusion would lead to indecision in areas where society demands decision.

PRODUCT OR REACTION

What are the distinguishing characteristics between behavior that is a direct *product of mental illness* and behavior that is in reaction to the illness? This is a special case of the allocation problem. It is more easily understood if the word *product* is used to mean feature or sign of the illness.

A person with pneumonia has certain signs and symptoms that are considered part and parcel of the illness. Fever, cough, chest pain, weakness and malaise, and white areas on X rays are all features of the disease, itself. Some who are hospitalized with pneumonia are model patients. They rest, ask for help only when they need it, are considerate of other patients and nursing staff, follow the prescribed regimen, etc. Others may resent being incapacitated. They will resist going to the hospital, be cantankerous, refuse to obey medical reccomendations, etc. Still others will find luxury in the incapacity. They will claim they are too weak to get out of bed when it would be good for them to do so, they will demand attention from visitors and staff, etc. These behaviors generally are not seen as features of pneumonia but rather as individual reactions to the illness. They stem from the healthy mental functions; they are chosen. The variety of ways people behave when they are sick is called *illness behavior* (Mechanic, 1962).

The situation with regard to mental illness is often less clear because behavior (even illness behavior) may be part of the illness per se. It is not quite so easy to distinguish between behavior that is a feature of the illness and that which is a reaction to it.

A thirty-two-year-old woman had been hospitalized for schizophrenia on numerous occasions. She would enter the hospital hallucinating with severe delusions of persecution. At these times, she would be convinced that her parents were impostors who were trying to imprison her for their own malicious, if mysterious, reasons.

The father was a wealthy industrialist who had very strong opinions. The mother was very conscious of the family's social position and reputation, and their daughter was an embarrassment to them. Years ago, the parents had sought out the best and most expensive treatment for the patient. She always responded to medication but sooner or later she discontinued it and her condition deteriorated. The family had become discouraged with the never-ending cycle of admission, improvement, discharge, and relapse.

During the periods when the patient was taking her medication, she acknowledged her parents but refused to live with them. She always suspected them of being ashamed of her and wanting to put her away at any opportunity. She felt awkward—a black sheep, inconsistent with the family's style of living. She was more comfortable living in a communal home with friends who were tolerant of her lack of sociability and occasional odd behavior.

Although the family had set up a trust fund for her, they were very disturbed by her style of living. They insisted that her lifestyle was a *product of mental illness,* and if she were not mentally ill, she could take her rightful place in the family and no one need be embarrassed. They would have preferred her remaining in the hospital to living in the commune.

Was this patient's style of living a feature of the illness or a reaction to it? Did it proceed from the sick mental functions or from the healthy ones? Was she driven to live in the commune or did she choose to?

On the one hand, whenever this woman went off her medication, the first sign of deterioration was withdrawal and increasing seclusiveness. Could it be that even at her best, on medication, she had an intolerance to socially stimulating situations? There is a category in DSM III (1980) called *residual schizophrenia,* which is characterized in part by relative social isolation. Perhaps, also, she was driven to avoid her parents by lingering, if unconscious, doubts about their valid claim to parenthood.

On the other hand, she knew her schizophrenia was an embarrassment to her family. Did she react to her illness by choosing to stay away? She knew the family would try to hospitalize her at the first sign of odd behavior. Did she decide on a safer place to live, given her condition and her family's attitude toward it?

In cases such as these, the individual has (or had) an illness, but what course should be taken with regard to the particular behavior in question? Should the behavior be excused as a manifestation of something beyond the patient's control, thus placing the individual in the sick role (Parsons, 1951)? Or is the mental illness acknowledged but the individual told he or she does not have to react that way to it; he or she can choose to act in a more desirable fashion — in an impaired role (Gordon, 1966)? One allocation will lead to an exemption from responsibility while the other will lead to assistance and exhortation to do better.

Psychiatric expertise is helpful in showing that the behavior in question is consistent with the mental illness, but when apportioning the allocation between sick influences and healthy (although perhaps undesirable) ones, nothing in a psychiatrist's training does or can prepare him or her for this task.

In summary, then, if psychiatrists can agree that a person is suffering from mental illness, the word *product* introduces its own complexities. In the practical world of decision making, society has taken certain philosophical positions which, while unprovable, seem to accord with common sense. It makes no practical difference whether a behavior was caused by the mental illness or was a feature of it. When the word *product* is used in this book, it refers to both viewpoints. In order to confront the questions asked by society, psychiatrists assume that ideas can cause actions with compelling force at times, while at other times they may provide a context in which a free choice or decision is made. Psychiatrists have no expertise in deciding which condition has occurred in any particular case.

A person can be partly mentally ill and partly well. In examining several areas of mental functioning, it may be found that some of these fit the criteria of illness while others do not. The problems in identifying clusters of mental characteristics as illness have been discussed in Chapter Two. The public at large is more ready to accept cognitive dysfunction as illness because it is qualitatively different from the thinking patterns employed by most people. However, emotion and urge characteristics differ only in degree or intensity from everyday experience, and these areas of functioning are less accepted as causes of a crippled choosing mechanism.

If these common sense assumptions of society are agreeable, then psychiatrists are faced with deciding whether a particular behavior was influenced by the sick part or the healthy part. This is the problem of allocation. That portion of the behavior allocated to the sick part is considered, by definition, to be inevitable or determined; it is a *product of mental illness.* That portion of the behavior allocated to the healthy part is considered to have been chosen in the context of the healthy ideas, emotions, etc.

In most decision-making situations, allocation takes place in two stages. It must first be decided if the behavior in question has been influenced by the sick part and/or the healthy part. In allocating to the sick part, psychiatrists identify the mentally ill characteristics and judge if the behavior is a reasonable outcome. This judgement requires no psychiatric expertise. The judgement is fortified, however, by noting if the behavior is consistent with that observed in people with the same diagnosis. This judgement is professional and requires psychiatrists to use their accumulated knowledge about the characteristics of various diagnostic categories.

In allocating to the healthy part, once again the test of reasonableness is applied. Is the behavior reasonably related to the context of ideas and emotions considered not ill? This judgement may be made by any reasonable person; it does not necessarily require a psychiatrist.

Following the first stage, often it is found that the behavior is allocated reasonably both to the sick and the healthy parts. The second stage consists in judging which part was more influential. Was the choosing mechanism overridden by illness or was it still sufficiently functional that the person had control over his or her behavior? No amount of expertise prepares a person to answer this question; it is a philosophical question, not a scientific one.

Thus, as with the concept of mental illness, the concept of *product* is exceedingly complex. While psychiatric expertise may play a small part, the really crucial questions society asks are matters about which psychiatrists can have no real expertise. When society or professional psychiatric activity confronts the *sick or _____?* questions, all of which are answered by the application of the *product of mental illness* formula, training and science fail; these are not questions of science but of philosophy and opinion. They are matters of policy. Psychiatrists have no expertise in answering the ultimate questions of either mental illness or *product.*

CHAPTER FOUR

THE DECISION PROCESS

P sychiatrists frequently must decide various *sick or* _____? questions that arise either in the course of practice or that are put to them by society. A substantial part of psychiatric decision making hinges on whether an individual's behavior is considered to be a *product of mental illness.* It is a bewildering task. While some people are undisputedly mentally ill, there are many who fall in the equivocal range. These are the tough decisions, the close calls that may give rise to vocal disagreement. Clinical facts and even laboratory data may illuminate the picture, but in the last analysis, whether a cluster of characteristics is labeled as a mental illness rests on policy decisions. Even if psychiatrists agree that a certain person suffers from mental illness, the problem exists of determining whether a particular behavior under scrutiny is a product of that illness. First, certain philosophical positions must be adopted, such as a libertarian framework and the view that sometimes ideas can cause behavior while at other times they merely may provide the context in which a free choice is made. These positions are matters of policy; there are no scientific guidelines that can make an expert in this area. In the cases where there is agreement that a person is suffering from mental illness, psychiatrists must allocate the behavior under scrutiny between the sick and the healthy parts of the individual. Their expertise here may be helpful, but it is not determinative. Weighing the balance between the sick and the healthy influences, the psychiatrist must decide whether the choosing mechanism was overcome and the individual was internally compelled to behave as he or she did. Again, there are no scientific guidelines for this balancing step; there is no expertise in this area.

Indeed, a dismal picture has been painted. It would seem that there is little in scientific or medical training that can prepare psychiatrists for many of the ultimate critical decisions they are called upon to make. Expert opinions would seem to be more opinion than expert. No one can have expertise when the ultimate questions are matters of opinion rather than fact. As such, the *sick or* _____? questions are issues of policy masquerading as issues of fact. When doctors ask, "Is this person sick or is he or she lazy?" they seem to be asking a fact question. When they ask, "Is the behavior a *product of mental illness?*" they seem to be inquiring about what the behavior is or is not. However, as was made so clear by Doctors Overholser and Duval, the questions really being asked are, "Should the person be called sick?" and "Should the behavior be allocated to a sick part of the individual?"

If the answers to these questions are matters of opinion, why does society continue to ask them? What is the sense of spending the considerable amount of time and money puzzling over questions, the answers to which depend on what people want to call it?

THE EMOTIONAL UNDERPINNING

This problem may be approached by examining a prediction made by Diamond (1962). He was concerned that despite the fact that Overholser and Duval (and other psychiatrists) had decided that sociopaths were mentally ill, the trend in the law was to exclude sociopathy from that group of conditions that qualified for the insanity defense. In other words, for a sociopath, the *sick or criminal?* question was likely to be decided in favor of criminal. Diamond said,

> So, at the risk of future mortification, I make the following predictions:
> 1. That within ten years, biochemical and physiological tests will be developed that will demonstrate beyond a reasonable doubt that a substantial number of our worst and most vicious criminal offenders are actually the sickest of all. And that if the concept of mental disease and exculpation from responsibility applies at all, it will apply equally to the vast horde of minor, habitual, aggressive offenders who form the great bulk of the recidivists. The law and the public, whether they like it or not, will be forced by the stark proof of scientific demonstration to accept the fact that large numbers of individuals who now receive the full, untempered blow of social indignation, ostracism, vengeance, and ritualized judicial murder

are sick and helpless victims of psychological and physical disease of the mind and brain. . . .

Suppose that there were such "stark proof of scientific demonstration." Would these facts impel society to treat the sociopathic, vicious criminal offenders as sick rather than criminal? Would this scientific demonstration save "the vast horde of minor habitual aggressive offenders" from "the full, untempered blow of social indignation, ostracism, vengeance and ritualized judicial murder?" In effect, Diamond predicted that scientific advances would prompt society to abandon the concept of criminality and to treat virtually all offenders as sick people.

Diamond was not the only psychiatrist to put forth the view that, given further advances in psychiatry, society would follow the rational path of treating rather than punishing. However, there is doubt whether all the scientific proof that might be mustered would ever lead to abandoning the concept of criminality and replacing it entirely with the concept of sickness. In the first place, as discussed in Chapter Two, basically, the concept of sickness rests on whether people feel the person could have acted differently if he or she wanted to. Science cannot answer the question of determinism versus libertarianism any more than it can answer the question of whether God created the heavens and the earth. And if a body of scientists claims to have sufficient proof to settle such questions, there will always be another body of people ready to scoff at such proof.

In the second place, even if scientists could convince the general public that criminals are really sick, and even if there were techniques by which these sick people could be treated, society would still not abandon its concept of criminality because rehabilitation of the offender is only one of society's goals. Society also seeks revenge and punishment. Victims demand satisfaction. Society simply does not want to replace "social indignation, ostracism, vengeance, and ritualized judicial murder" with scientific help for the offender. In other words, the hope that society would substitute rational reactions for its emotional ones will not be realized because emotions run high in criminal cases. (Hart [1958] emphasized the importance of the need for vengeance and retribution. Goldstein [1967, p. 15], discussing the goals of the criminal law, said that "underlying all, as the single constant element is the concept of blame.") Society demands justice and, as Kelsen (1953) has emphasized, emotions are important in deciding what is just. And Judge Bazelon, after struggling with the concept of *product of mental illness* for almost twenty years after he wrote the *Durham* opinion, finally decided that the *sick or criminal?* question should be decided on the basis of whether the jury felt that the defendant "can justly be held responsible" (*United States u Brawner,* 1972, Bazelon, J., partial dissent). In other words, the decision should be based on the jury's sense of justice—how it feels about the situation.

If the emotions underlying blame are so powerful, why pose the *sick or criminal?* question altogether? Why not blame every offender? This question will be dealt with more extensively in Chapter Six. At this point, note that the concept of justice requires exceptions— circumstances where society feels it would be wrong to blame. One of these exceptions is sickness. If psychiatrists decide the person could not help him or herself, how can society blame? Helplessness engenders another emotion—compassion. The desire to hurt some-one changes to a desire to help. Indeed, the emotion of compas-sion underlies the concept of sickness in all the *sick or* _____? situations.

One reason the *product* questions must be asked is that they deal with very strong emotions. For example, when the *"sick or criminal?"* question is asked, society must also ask if the course of action is based primarily on outrage and fear (the underpinnings of blame) or primarily on compassion. Tensions between other emotions form the bedrock of other *sick or* _____? questions.

Human beings have a wide repertoire of emotions. They come in all shades and hues—intense and muted, obvious and subtle. This book shall deal only with four of them, and two of them will be condensed into one. This is a gross oversimplification, but it makes the discussion manageable. The emotional components of *product of mental illness* decisions are outrage and fear, compassion, and indifference. Outrage may be minimal, as in annoyance; moderate, as in disgust; or severe, as in fury. It may be mixed with fear. Although the emotion of fear is different from that of the anger found in pure outrage, the effect in terms of society's deci-sions is often the same. People try to put distance between themselves and those for whom they have either outrage or fear. They blame the individual for the behavior in question whether they are angry at him or her or whether they are afraid. Therefore, for further simplification, fear will be included as a component of outrage.

Compassion evokes more of an attitude of approaching the other person rather than avoiding him or her as in the case of outrage. It may vary from an understanding of the other individual's position to a mild sympathy or a strong, caretaking devotion.

No one is ever completely indifferent to another individual, but humans are quite often relatively indifferent. They take the position that "it is none of my business," or "it doesn't really matter to me what happens to him or her." Indifference should not be confused with not wanting personally to intervene. One may keep oneself aloof from a situation while still having strong feelings that someone else should do something about it.

Outrage and compassion, with indifference as the relative absence of either, are basic to group living. Given any individual's behavior, the emotional reaction it will evoke from others will vary according to several factors. Dangerous behavior tends to provoke outrage; helpless behavior, compassion. Whether the behavior is perceived as dangerous or helpless may vary with teachings of each particular culture. Some societies and some periods of history seem to emphasize outrage, while others emphasize compassion and indifference. Within any one culture, different individuals, whether out of timidity, the need to maintain self-esteem, guilt, or countless other personal themes, will react with different emotions to any particular behavior under scrutiny. But the important fact is that they will react. No human society is or can be without emotion. And furthermore, despite the variations in the types and degrees of emotional response, every culture and every human group must have some expressions of outrage (including the fear component), compassion, and indifference.

These emotions are part of human biology. At the very least, humans could not react with outrage, compassion, and indifference if these emotional states were not built into their repertoires. They are part of the equipment with which people are born. Beyond this, they are essential components for the maintenance of society. For example, the compassion elicited by the helpless behavior of infants promotes parental caretaking. The outrage felt when family, friends, or community are attacked are crucial to the protection of the group. Even indifference is important to society. People need their own private time. They must protect themselves from an excess of emotional involvements. Disengagement from intense relationships serves two functions: It gives the opportunity, within limits, for people to do what they want and to develop somewhat independently from the group, and it frees others from being so concerned about one person that they cannot attend to other needs of the group.

Sociobiologists such as Wilson (1975) have concluded that many social behavior patterns are programed by the genes of that particular species in order to maximize conditions so that the species may reproduce. Van den Berghe (1977, p. 44) has observed that various animals "tend to favor kin over non-kin and favor close kin over distant kin." There seem to be biological mechanisms encouraging people to protect the welfare of those close to them in preference to those who are distant and dissimilar. These mechanisms seem to be part of human genetic heritage. It is not difficult to surmise that compassion is one such mechanism that fosters the survival of kin and close group members, while outrage is more likely to be vented toward strangers.

This implies that through the ages, compassion, outrage, and indifference have been indelibly bred into the human species. These emotions are fundamental building blocks in the biology of human social groups. The way these emotions are expressed may vary from group to group and from situation to situation; however, no human group can exist without these emotions any more than it can exist without hunger and sexuality.

There are various ways of classifying deviant people, as discussed in Chapter One. They can be referred to as sick, criminal, sinful, unwise, lazy, manipulative, unpleasant, or inexperienced. Except for the sick and inexperienced, all are held responsible for their actions. Even if society may have some compassion for them, people feel "It is their own fault." Society will react primarily with outrage or indifference. Only the sick and the inexperienced could not have behaved better.

While it is felt that the sick and the inexperienced could not help themselves, there is a basic difference between them. The helplessness of the inexperienced comes from the outside while the helplessness of the sick comes from within. The inexperienced person is perfectly able to choose but lacks having had the outside experiences necessary to choose wisely. The sick person is crippled from within. And of these two classes, it is only the sick classification that poses such difficult philosophical questions about determinism and libertarianism.

In other words, all the deviant classifications except sick are predicated on the assumption that the individual has an intact choosing mechanism. Of all the deviant behaviors, only mental illness assumes that the choosing mechanism is overridden by compelling internal causes. Society justly cannot hold a mentally ill person responsible for his or her actions. Nor can the situation be remedied by teaching, as with inexperience. The mentally sick person evokes a maximum of compassion and must be healed. Or is it the other way around?

I suggest that the deviant behavior initially evokes compassion and that this feeling causes people to decide that the person is sick and to allocate to the sick part the greater influence on the choosing mechanism. In the last analysis, then, the subtle philosophical questions raised in the preceding two chapters are resolved on the basis of how people *feel* about the individual in question. When it comes particularly to the close calls about whether a person is mentally ill, it is compassion or the lack of it which makes people decide that the behavior under scrutiny is a *product of mental illness.*

Because some degree of outrage will always exist in human society, some people always will be held responsible for their deviant behavior. Because some degree of compassion will always exist in human society, some people always will be exempt from responsibility for their deviant behavior. Because outrage, compassion, and indifference are inevitably part of the biology of human social relationships, there will always be *sick or* _____? questions. This is why so much time and money are spent pursuing the *product of mental illness* question—a question the answers to which depend on opinion, on how society *feels.* People must ask these questions; they are the moral and cognitive counterparts to basic emotional tugs. They are a part of being human.

To recapitulate, if, *product of mental illness* questions ultimately cannot be decided on the basis of fact, why does society persist in asking these questions? Close examination reveals that strong emotions of outrage (which include fear), compassion, and indifference underlie decisions in the *Sick or* _____? questions. The circumstances that evoke each of these emotions may vary from person to person and from culture to culture. However, these emotions are basic to the maintenance of all human social groups, and they are part of the sociobiological heritage. Because no human society can exist without these emotions and their intellectual derivatives, the *product of mental illness* questions,. in some form or other, must be asked. People ask them because they are human.

THE INTELLECTUAL OVERLAY

If the *product* questions fundamentally are decided by the way humans feel, should the *sick or* _____? questions be put to decision makers in that form? Judge Bazelon substantially proposed this over a decade ago when he suggested that the jury base its decision on what it felt was just. The proposal met with no enthusiasm, however, and courts and legislatures have continued to seek some intellectual methods for resolving the *sick or* _____? questions.

One reason intellectual guidelines are sought, of course, is that human beings are not only emotional creatures; they have ideas as well. Every society has a need for orderliness and predictability (Bodenheimer, 1974, Chapter 10). If decisions can be made willy-nilly, there will be no societal institutions. Civilized society must have rules and laws to inform people what to expect in various situations.

Leaving the matter in each individual case up to the decision-maker would be both too whimsical and too unpredictable. If the referee or judge were in a grumpy mood, the unlucky petitioner would be treated with little compassion; if the decisionmaker had just been given a surprise office party, more compassion might be shown. In point of fact, because of human nature this does occur to some degree, but the intellectual guidelines for decision making are an attempt to reduce the amount of this capriciousness.

Then, too, the various *product* questions arise in many different contexts, as described in Chapter One. In each situation, if the decision is made that the individual's behavior is a *product of mental illness,* one form of action is taken; if not, another form is taken. These contexts are so different from each other that society may have different emotional tugs regarding them. For example, society may wish to insure that more compassion is shown toward people when putting them in mental hospitals than is shown when giving them excuses for missing work. In other words, the community has considerable stake in deciding the *product* questions in each context. Intellectual guidelines can help tilt the balance of the decision toward society's goal in each situation.

Nonetheless, it is this intellectual overlay that also causes the *product* dilemma. If human beings were content merely to react with outrage, compassion, or indifference, there would be no logical problem. But when emotional reactions are applied to the decision situation, humans are impelled either to hold the person responsible for his or her actions or to exempt him or her from responsibility. This is the libertarian position that was described in Chapter Two. Society believes that most people can choose their actions except when they are mentally ill. As Justice Cardozo states, "[The law] is guided by a robust common sense which assumes the freedom of the will as a working hypothesis in the solution of legal problems" (*Steward Machine Co. v. Davis,* 1937). Psychiatrists asked to participate in this decision process have been trained in a deterministic mode; their expertise fails them when they are asked if an individual could choose freely.

In almost every *product* situation, there are three stages in the decision process: the competing societal interests, the guidelines for resolving the *sick or _____?* questions, and the decision in the individual case. Each of these stages can be expressed in terms of ideas, rules, procedures, etc. These comprise the intellectual overlay. However, at their crucial points, each stage rests on an emotional base reflecting tension between compassion and outrage or compassion and indifference. The dilemmas of *product* arise as the decision process demands there be a leap from the determinism of psychiatry to the libertarian position demanded by society's robust common sense. Somehow these dilemmas must be resolved.

STAGE ONE—COMPETING SOCIETAL INTERESTS. Behind every *sick or _____?* question lie competing interests and aims of society. Should society compel certain people to go to mental hospitals or should it allow everyone to make up his or her own mind? Once a business contract is signed, should people be held responsible for their actions if they were mentally ill and did not know what they were doing? There are powerful arguments on both sides that represent the various goals of society. There are many such interests, often in conflict with each other (Feeley, 1976). Some are rarely articulated but remain as powerful hidden agendas.

Often, these interests are expressed in terms of rights—the right to liberty, the right to equal opportunity, etc. Where do these rights come from? They come from people, individually and collectively, although they may be attributed to God and nature as well (Rand, 1965). These rights, which form the cornerstones upon which laws and court decisions are built, are expressions of cultural values—the way people *feel* about things. For example, in American society, freedom from government intervention is a highly valued right; in totalitarian societies, the government's right to command cooperation and order is more highly valued.

People tend to think that rights are absolute, but despite the ringing rhetoric of the Declaration of Independence that all people "are endowed by their Creator with certain unalienable Rights," no rights are "unalienable." Whenever there is a clash between different rights, whenever there are competing societal aims and interests, any right may be subject to modification or abridgement.

Society's interests and aims are shaped by many forces, such as historical precedent, religious preferences, political ideologies, economics, etc. The policymakers of society, the judges, legislators, and administrators who set up the guidelines for resolving the *sick or _____?* questions must weigh and balance the various competing societal interests. When they weigh the importance of the various interests, they must consider not only the historical precedents but also the current social climate—the temper of the times. For example, in the 1950s, many enlightened and educated people felt a wave of optimism that psychiatry, sociology, and a host of other disciplines dealing with human behavior were on the verge of providing scientific solutions to pressing social problems. Psychoanalytic thinking had become part of the popular culture and it seemed that previously inexplicable behavior would soon become understandable in terms of causes and effects. This period saw an upsurge in compassion. The policymakers tended to broaden the criteria of *product* so that more and more behavior could be seen as resulting from mental illness. In the 1970s, the rights of individuals to be free from government intervention came to the fore and policymakers made it more difficult to label behavior as *products of mental illness*, which justified involuntary hospitalization. The balance was tipped toward indifference. In the early 1980s, outrage about crime was mounting and the policymakers were responding by attempting to make it more difficult for people to qualify for the insanity defense.

Society is a dynamic, moving and breathing organism, and the balance of competing interests made by the policymakers, representing what society feels is fair and just, changes with its movements. As society moves through successive periods of greater outrage, compassion, or indifference, with consequent swings in the value policymakers give to the various competing societal interests, the guidelines (stage two) set by the policymakers change back and forth. Harper and Kime (1934) have referred to the elasticity of the law as it molds itself to the temper of the times.

For this reason, society should not expect rigid, lasting cookbook guidelines for deciding *product* questions. Legal history will repeat itself over and over as the balance of the competing societal interests tilts first in one direction and then in another in response to the temper of the times.

What role should psychiatrists play as society balances the competing social interests? They should inform the public and the policymakers about the system for delivering treatment to the mentally ill, their needs, and the degree to which psychiatric personnel are available. They might comment on some anticipated consequences of a change in the balance of competing interests, such as the fact that a strong tilt toward compassion might necessitate a larger budget for mental health services. Issues such as these are well within the realm of their professional expertise and require no shift from the deterministic framework of science to the libertarian viewpoint of society. However, in their professional roles, they should not pretend to any special knowledge about how the balance of the competing societal interests should result. The tilt toward outrage, compassion, or indifference is not a psychiatric question; it is a matter of social policy. There is no psychiatric expertise that can enable them to tell the policymakers which of the competing interests is more important than the others (Hartmann, 1960; Bursten, 1974).

STAGE TWO—GUIDELINES. After society's policymakers balance the competing interests, they promulgate guidelines in the form of laws or rules to be followed when *Sick or* _____? cases must be decided. If the balance tilts toward compassion, the guidelines will be formulated in such a way that more people will be designated sick; if the balance tilts toward outrage or indifference, the rules will nudge more people into the criminal, unwise, etc. categories.

For convenience, in this discussion the two types of guidelines are separated—procedures and standards. Procedures describe the process that must be observed when a particular case is to be decided. Standards spell out the definition of what the policymakers wish to label as sick behavior in each situation.

Procedures include such issues as whether the individual has a right to an attorney, whether there must be a formal hearing, whether there is a right to an appeal, etc. They spell out who must prove the case—the one claiming sickness or the one claiming not sickness. While these procedures are of considerable importance and are often the subject of intense debate, little space shall be devoted to them in this book because they do not directly involve the problems of psychiatric expertise in determining which behavior is a *product of mental illness.*

The standards are the guidelines that speak directly to the dilemma of *product.* The standards spell out the criteria that must be used in order to designate a particular behavior as a *product of mental illness.* (1) Generally, they require the person to have a mental illness at the time of the behavior in question. (2) They may be even more specific and require that the illness must have been manifested by certain mental characteristics, such as types of cognition, emotion, and/or urge. (3) They always require that the behavior in question has resulted from (be a product of) the mental illness in 1 and, where applicable, the specific mental characteristics in 2.

The standards define a circle. Individuals falling within the circle are to be treated as sick; those falling outside the circle are to be treated as criminal, unwise, etc. If the policymakers tilt toward compassion, they will include many conditions within the circle. If they tilt toward outrage or indifference, the circle will include fewer conditions.

When the elements of standard are examined, the product dilemma is immediately confronted. The first requirement is that the individual must have a mental illness. But, as seen in Chapter Two, who is to say which clusters of mental characteristics are illness and which are not? It is easy enough for society's policymakers to set up mental illness as a requirement, but how can the decisionmaker in stage three decide whether a particular person under scrutiny meets this standard? Certainly, psychiatric expertise cannot be decisive.

There is a possible way out of this dilemma. The standard of *mentally ill* could be changed to *sufficiently mentally ill.* Many different types of people could be included within the category of sufficient mental illness; there would not be a need to distinguish between the mentally ill and the nonill. The policymakers would be saying, "Of all the types and degrees of mental illness that people might argue about, for the purpose of this standard, only these types and these degrees will be considered sufficiently mentally ill to be included within the circle." Note that the word *sufficiently* changes the thrust of the question from a policy issue to a factual one.

One of the advantages of the new psychiatric nomenclature (DSM III) is that each diagnostic category has reasonably specific criteria. It is not a perfect system; there is still room for disagreement among psychiatrists with regard to an individual's diagnosis. However, there is every reason to expect that on important classes of illness, the reliability of psychiatric diagnosis will be higher than previously. The policymakers could designate certain diagnostic categories as sufficient mental illness. Those people who have different diagnoses would lie outside the circle regardless of how ill they might seem. Those diagnostic categories that are considered sufficiently mentally ill will be referred to as *threshold mental illnesses*, because if the individual under scrutiny in stage three does not have one of them, the decisionmaker need not go any further. For the purposes of this particular decision, the behavior cannot be a *product of mental illness.*

How can society's policymakers know which diagnostic categories they wish to include within the circle? Prompted by the balance of competing societal interests, they will have compassion for certain kinds of people, but what do they know about the diagnostic categories? Here is where the psychiatrists come in; their expertise lies in diagnosis. The process of leaping from the expertise of diagnosis to society's expression of compassion is *transduction* (Bursten, 1982a). Transduction is the process by which information in one system actuates information in a different system. For example, the electrical information from the wires in a telephone actuates the mechanical information of sound waves (transduction) that actuates the auditory information in the listener (transduction).

Psychiatrists use their expertise to describe the thought processes, feelings, and behaviors characteristic of each diagnostic category. This can be done without leaving the deterministic mode so long as psychiatrists do not refer to inhibition of the ability to choose. The societal policymakers receiving this information can perform the transduction by considering if this is the kind of person that society, in its robust common sense, feels should be able to control his or her choices, or if it feels that such a person could not help him or herself. In other words, given the diagnostic description by the psychiatrists, the policymakers react on the basis of outrage or indifference on the one hand or compassion on the other. Those categories that arouse the policymakers' compassion would be considered sufficiently mentally ill to lie within the circle.

The role of the psychiatrists is to inform, not to advise. Policymakers can be given the information they need, but they should not pretend any expertise in deciding which diagnosis should be included within the circle.

One might argue that such a process for setting up standards is too complex and cumbersome. However, it is already being done, both formally and haphazardly. The formal process is found, for example, in certain standards for the judgement of criminal responsibility. Voluntary intoxication usually does not qualify as a threshold diagnosis for the insanity defense (*Hopt v People*, 1881) and narcotic addiction has been specifically excluded in *United States v Freeman* (1966). In essence, the policymakers have decided that these conditions are not sufficient mental illnesses. However, the policymakers should specify which diagnoses lie within rather than outside of the circle of threshold illnesses.

The haphazard process usually occurs in stage three of the decision process rather than in stage two. Given the ambiguous standard of mental illness, the decisionmaker listens to the psychiatric testimony about an individual and rather informally says, "That's not what we mean by crazy!"

In addition to setting up threshold diagnoses, the policymakers may wish further to limit the variety of conditions lying within the circle by specifying certain cognitive, emotional, or urge features. Thus, for example, in criminal cases, only that paranoid schizophrenia with a misunderstanding of the wrongfulness of the action might count; paranoid schizophrenia with an intensification of anger would not be sufficient. Once again, this criterion would reflect the degree of compassion the policymakers had when they balanced the competing societal interests. The role of the psychiatrists in setting up this standard, as before, would be to inform, not to advise. The policymakers need to know which cognitive, emotional, and urge characteristics are features of the diagnostic categories they have selected. It is well within the expertise of psychiatrists to give them this information.

The third element of the standards is that the behavior in question be a product of the threshold mental illness, as defined by the diagnostic categories and, where applicable, by the specific mental characteristics. This element goes into the standards automatically. It requires no decision on the part of society's policymakers and its inclusion in the standards poses no *product* dilemma at this point. However, it creates serious problems in stage three when the individual case must be decided.

STAGE THREE—DECIDING THE INDIVIDUAL CASE. The essential task in stage three of the decision process is to ascertain whether any particular case fits the standards. If the standards remain as they are currently, with mental illness as the criterion, either of two impossible situations arise. (1) The psychiatrist must specify whether the individual in question is mentally ill—an impossible task. (2) Society's decisionmaker (e.g. a judge or jury) must decide if there is mental illness. Since mental illness is a matter of social policy resting on compassion, this course does not seem unreasonable. However, it becomes awkward because the decisionmaker usually wants to rely on the psychiatrist. If the psychiatrist states that a person has an intermittent explosive disorder with subtle deviations on sophisticated neuropsychological tests, and society's decisionmaker says, "That's not what I mean by crazy!" it would seem that the layperson is trying to outdiagnose the doctor. A much more orderly and predictable course, and one that avoids the appearance of lay diagnosis, can occur if the criterion of sufficient mental illness previously outlined is adopted. In this situation, the psychiatrist, using his or her expertise, could state whether the person meets one of the threshold diagnoses. Where specific mental characteristics have been added to the criteria, the psychiatrist could state whether the person shows these particular cognitive, emotional, or urge characteristics and whether they are features of the diagnostic category in question.

It is when the third element of the standards—that the behavior is a product of the threshold mental illness—is confronted that again the *product* dilemma is met. Here arises the problem of allocation of the behavior in question between the sick and healthy aspects of the individual. This has been discussed in detail in Chapter Three. Whether the choosing mechanism was crippled by the (threshold) sick influences about which the psychiatrist has testified or whether the person could have withstood these influences is a question clearly phrased in the libertarian "robust common sense" of society rather than in the deterministic framework of psychiatric expertise. Once again, a transduction is necessary. Some decisionmaker must take the facts given by the psychiatrist (and perhaps others) about the person's sufficiently sick influences together with the facts given by the witnesses about characteristics not reasonably related to threshold illnesses and weigh them. These facts will activate the decisionmaker's outrage, compassion, or indifference and he or she will decide whether that the individual's choosing mechanism was crippled. This is the manner in which the *sick or* _____? questions are answered. The facts activate systems that produce opinions; information gathered in the deterministic context is transduced into the libertarian context.

An example might help make stage three of the decision process clearer. For the insanity defense, assume the standard lists senile dementia as a threshold diagnosis. Sufficient mental illness is further limited by the specific mental characteristic of a misunderstanding of the wrongfulness of the situation. Emotionality and urge are disallowed as criteria.

A seventy-five-year-old man displayed increasing suspiciousness and irritability. As his memory became affected and he began to misplace things, he started to accuse his wife of stealing his possessions and his money. Like many people with this illness, he had some better days when his memory improved and he was more reasonable.

This man's relationship with his wife had been poor for many years prior to the onset of his dementia. He had a deep contempt for her and he frequently had expressed the wish that she would "go away or die or something." The wife, for her part, had the knack of saying the wrong thing at the wrong time; she could be very provocative. He had hit her in anger on many occasions.

On the night in question, he shot her with his rifle. Then, he went out on the porch and sat in his rocking chair until morning when he was found by his son who had stopped by on the way to work. The old man gave several different statements to the police and the examining psychiatrist. "I don't remember it—is she really dead?" "Good riddance!" "Sure I shot her, she was stealing me blind. Nothing wrong with that, not when you shoot a thief in your own house." "Serves her right, the old crow!"

The psychiatrist could testify that the defendant met the criteria for a threshold mental illness—senile dementia. There was some evidence that he failed to comprehend the wrongfulness of his

actions and that this misunderstanding was related to the suspiciousness which is a feature of senile dementia. He made no
attempt to leave the scene or hide the weapon. Even the fact that
the incident happened at night is consistent with the threshold
mental illness because people with senile dementia may become
particularly confused at night.

On the other hand, the psychiatrist and other witnesses could
have noted the history of physical violence that antedated the
dementia. Some of the defendant's statements after the shooting
indicate no confusion at all, but rather considerable satisfaction.

All of these facts could be presented to the jury. These facts were
based on observation and expertise. The jury, using the "robust
common sense" of the society whose representative it is, makes the
transduction. The jurors weigh the sick aspects against the healthy
ones, have their compassion or their outrage stirred, and designate the defendant as sick or criminal. How would you, the reader,
decide? Is your decision not based on your feeling of "This poor
man"—compassion, or "This nasty man; we can't let these people
get away with it"—outrage? Remember, a choice must be made.

What is proposed then, is that in deciding the individual
case, society must make the transduction through its designated
representatives. They are the people who are chosen to represent
the "robust common sense" of the society from which they are
drawn. These representatives will vary from situation to situation.
This proposal allows the psychiatrist to stay within the realm of
his or her expertise. There may be times, however, when it may be
expedient to use the psychiatrist not only as an expert but also as a
representative of society. Psychiatrists, too, are products of a culture and can reflect its values and opinions. If they are put in this
dual role, they clearly should stipulate where their professional
expertise ends and their role as a representative of society begins.

Thus, a one-transduction procedure for stage three has been
proposed. The psychiatrist speaks in terms of his or her expertise,
other witnesses may present facts, and society's representatives
make the transduction that decides the *product* question. It is also
possible to have a two-transduction procedure; actually this occurs
in many criminal trials. Often the psychiatrist is asked if the
patient has met the criteria set forth in the insanity standards. The

psychiatrist may say, for example, "In my opinion, the defendant, because of mental illness, substantially was not able to conform his behavior to the requirements of law." The jury, then weighing all the testimony, reaches its own conclusion. Regardless of what the psychiatrist has testified, it is the jury that makes the ultimate transduction and decides the issue (*Washington u United States*, 1967).

There may even be an advantage to the two-transduction procedure in stage three. The psychiatrist is very knowledgeable about the medical aspects of the situation; this is his or her area of expertise. As previously noted, the psychiatrist is also a representative of society's views, but he or she may be unduly biased toward compassion. It might be said that the psychiatrist has high expertise in the deterministic framework of medicine but a relatively low expertise in the libertarian framework of society's expectations.

The situation with the jury is (at least theoretically) just the reverse. Society has designated these people to reflect its values: It has high expertise in the libertarian framework of "robust common sense." On the other hand, the jury has low expertise in the data of medicine.

Thus, the two transductions tend to complement each other. By analogy, consider that there are certain words in Chinese that have no exact counterpart in German. If a person wishes to render one such word and in its concept in German and if there is a Chinese scholar and a German scholar, each of whom knows something about the other's language, the use of both services may be desirable.

The intellectual overlay will be reviewed. Human beings are driven to pose *sick or* _____? questions by the powerful emotions of outrage, compassion, and indifference. Order and predictability are given to the solutions of these questions through a three stage decision process. Society's policymakers wittingly and unwittingly weigh and balance the various competing interests and goals of society. As the emotional temper of the times changes back and forth, the balance of these interests tilts more toward outrage, compassion, or indifference.

Stage two involves the setting up of guidelines for the resolu-

tion of the *sick or* _____? questions in the various situations in
which they arise. While there are many procedures that govern
whether society will show more or less compassion—whether greater
or fewer numbers of people will be designated as sick—this book
primarily will be concerned with the standards that attempt to
define who will be treated compassionately. It has been suggested
that these standards be predicated on the concept of sufficient
mental illness—a concept that would include certain diagnostic
categories and perhaps certain specific cognitive, emotive, and/or
urge characteristics. The process by which society's policymakers
arrive at what is to be sufficient mental illness requires a transduction. They are given descriptions of the diagnoses and characteristics by psychiatrists and, prompted by their emotional responses,
they select some of them to be included within the circle of
sufficient illness. These are the threshold mental illnesses. Every
standard also requires the behavior under scrutiny to be a product
of the illnesses within the circle.

Stage three involves seeing if the individual case fits the standards.
Psychiatrists can testify within the area of their expertise about
whether the individual has a threshold mental illness. It is society's
representatives, however, that should allocate the behavior in
question between the sick and healthy aspects of the individual.
Prompted by all the testimony, these representatives react emotionally and transduce the facts into "robust common sense." They
are the ones who ultimately determine if a particular behavior is a
product of mental illness.

CHAPTER FIVE

MALINGERING

A three-stage process has been described for deciding whether behavior is a *product of mental illness:* The balance of competing societal interests, the setting up of standards (and procedures, that will not be considered in this book), and the decision of whether the individual case meets these standards.

Doctors often are called upon to testify whether an individual meets the criteria for a particular illness in the realm of their specialty. And this is precisely what psychiatrists are asked to do in stage three. Whether the standards stipulate mental illness as they do currently, or sufficient mental illness as has been proposed, the person must be evaluated and the psychiatrist must testify whether he or she meets the criteria for certain diagnoses and particular mental characteristics. However, the task is often more difficult than that of other specialists because psychiatrists are dealing with mental characteristics, which by their very nature are not directly observable. For example, if a person is told to move his or her arm and the arm remains motionless, the neurologist can apply certain tests to determine if there are dysfunctions of the nerves and muscles. If there is no physiological problem, there are still several psychiatric possibilities. It may be that the individual anticipates pain and is afraid to move the arm (psychogenic pain). It may be that he or she is convinced the arm is paralyzed and feels no power to move it (conversion disorder). Or it may be that the person knows he or she can move the arm but for a variety of reasons prefers to pretend that he or she cannot (malingering).

Often the behavior in question involves action rather than nonmovement. For example, if a person sets a fire, a diagnosis cannot be made until it is known whether the person felt that "voices" made him or her do it or he or she believed that the action

83

was the only way to counteract some malicious plot (possibly paranoid schizophrenia). If the person seems to have lost ambition and sociability after an automobile accident (and there is no evidence of brain damage), the presence of nightmares, rumination about the accident, feelings of numbness, etc. can help differentiate between post-traumatic stress disorder and faking in order to collect more insurance.

In all of these examples, whether the patient meets the criteria set up by the stage two standards depends on his or her inner experiences. Psychiatrists become aware of them only as they are reported, and unfortunately, reports of inner experiences can be faked. In many of the situations discussed in this book, it may be to the individual's advantage to lie about what he or she is experiencing.

Since the problem of faking or malingering can bedevil *product of mental illness* decisions, it should be confronted at this juncture. Malingering commonly is conceptualized as the voluntary production of symptoms (Boydston, 1980). This may include both behaviors that simulate illness and reports of inner experiences consistent with illness. This way of viewing malingering implies that sick behavior is compelled (nonvoluntary) while malingered behavior is chosen. Again, the determinism-libertarianism morass may engulf us. Suppose the attribute of voluntariness is changed to "a feeling of voluntariness." People are aware that they feel in control of some actions, but others feel compelled and beyond their control. Malingering, then, occurs when the person feels that he or she is purposely simulating the symptoms that are displayed or reported; if the person feels that the symptoms are beyond his or her control, there is no malingering. In this discussion, *simulation* will be referred to rather than *the feeling of simulation* in order to render the wording less awkward.

While this conceptualization clears up a philosophical difficulty, a serious methodological problem is still left. How can someone know what another person actually feels? A psychiatrist must rely on "nothing more infallible than one man's assessment of what is going on in another man's mind" (Miller, 1969).

Generally, two types of data are employed in the evaluation of malingering; psychiatrists assess whether the entire symptom pattern is consistent with those mental characteristics that comprise a diagnostic category and they try to gain some insight into how generally truthful and reliable a character the individual has.

Psychiatric expertise may be helpful in detecting malingering because certain characteristics go together to make up a mental illness. Sometimes the symptoms that are presented just do not make sense. For example, one very inept malingerer claimed he heard voices. When asked if he usually saw yellow lights off to the left when he heard the voices. he replied, "Yes, right over there," and he pointed to the left. When questioned further if he suffered from cramps on the right side of his stomach after he saw the yellow lights, he responded, "Right here, right here," and pointed to his right side.

Most often malingering is not quite that obvious. A man who was accused of rape insisted he had no memory of the event. He did not deny having done it; he just could not remember. He insisted he was not crazy; he did not hear voices or feel that people were conspiring against him. He just suffered from memory lapse. He seemed quite cooperative in the interview. In fact, his hands shook with tension as he tried to remember. He stated that the memory lapse made him "very nervous."

This was not a total amnesia. He knew his name, but not where he worked or what his occupation was. He could remember his father's name, but not the city where he was raised. He could not recall how far he had gone in school.

This condition started immediately after he had been identified by the victim. She knew him, and she and other witnesses reported no amnesia prior to the date of the offense. It had now been several months since he had been jailed and the amnesia had not changed.

The spottiness of the memory difficulty, especially with regard to events long preceding the incident in question was not typical of amnesias. The unchanging character of the memory loss with no recovery over several months was also atypical. The dramatic display of tension as the defendant tried to remember seemed overdone in comparison with the expressions of confusion that people with amnesia often show. In other words, the collection of characteristics that were reported and displayed did not fit reasonably the cluster characteristic of a mental illness—psychogenic amnesia. A psychiatric expert did not have to call the person a liar or even diagnose him as a malingerer; the only conclusion to be drawn was that he did not exhibit the characteristics of a threshold illness.

Of course, when reaching that conclusion, psychiatrists usually do imply that the individual was simulating. A doctor cannot know whether the patient was voluntarily producing the symptoms; this can be inferred only from the evidence. In the case of the so-called amnesiac, this inference was supported by the fact that after the interview, he walked back to his cell. When he realized he was being observed, he started to stagger.

In evaluating the consistency of the mental characteristics, there are six areas that should be considered.

1. The symptoms of the illness are the thoughts and feelings reported by the person. These, of course, easily can be simulated.

2. Signs of an illness are directly observable by others. Many signs easily can be faked. The psychiatrist can ask the person to remember three items and the individual can say, "I don't remember." Or, the person may give the wrong month and year when asked for the date. These may be signs of recent memory loss or orientation difficulty, but they also may be simulations. What the psychiatrist must look for here is the consistency of the signs and symptoms with a diagnostic cluster of characteristics.

3. Certain signs are not easily faked. Emotional display that is widely disparate from what is being talked about, speech that has a pressured, propulsive quality, specific disturbances of syntax such as spinning off in all directions or jumping from subject to subject in the middle of a thought are very difficult to imitate in a convincing fashion. It is rare that these signs are simulated. A competent psychiatrist usually can detect these signs and count them as not simulated.

4. Laboratory data usually cannot be simulated.

5. The individual may report certain limitations of activities. Again, this report may not reflect his or her actual activities. It is very easy for the person to claim that he or she rarely goes visiting

because people make him or her uneasy, but this report may be inaccurate.

6. The verification of the activities report given by the patient is crucial. It is important to know if the reported signs disappear when the doctor leaves, because this is not characteristic of mental illnesses. The reports of people who witness the patient at other times may be helpful, except when they, too, may have a stake in the success of the deception. Reports of previous hospitalizations are particularly useful. In this area, psychiatric expertise may be of less importance than good detective work. The psychiatrist is well advised to make ample use of this detective work in order to assess whether the symptom pattern really fits the threshold mental illness. If the psychiatrist diagnoses a conversion disorder on the basis of a patient's inability to move his or her legs, and other witnesses have moving pictures of the patient riding a bicycle, society's representatives may be justified in wresting the power of making the diagnosis from the psychiatrist.

On occasion, especially in child abuse, custody, and personal injury cases, attorneys deliberately have withheld information that would have branded their clients as neglectful or even dangerous parents. Despite request for all information, they justify withholding information on the grounds that they do not want to prejudice the evaluation of a psychiatrist. Therefore, it is necessary for those who testify to use wording such as, "On the basis of the information available to me and if there is no countervailing information, my opinion is. . . . " In this way, in the cross-examination if new information becomes available, the testimony of the psychiatrist cannot be discredited.

Psychiatric expertise is useful particularly in detecting the signs in the interview that cannot be faked easily and in knowing if all the signs and symptoms add up to a known cluster of mental characteristics. The signs that are not faked easily are those chiefly belonging to the psychoses. Frequently, however, the complaint falls in a diagnostic category that does not include such signs (see Chapter Eight). Conversion disorders, psychogenic pain, anxieties, and personality changes, as features of massive stress or head injuries, all must rely for diagnosis on symptoms and reports of changes in activity level. No special psychiatric expertise is needed or helpful here; only good detective work can confirm a diagnosis of malingering.

Davidson (1965) has suggested psychiatrists also assess the character of the patient. For example, a diagnosis of malingering is supported by a past history of irresponsibility or lying, shying away from medical examinations, and an unwillingness to try other forms of employment that would not involve his or her symptoms. In other words, is this the kind of person who is likely to be trying to get away with something? One example of the usefulness of behavior and characterological attributes in ruling out malingering was presented by a plaintiff evaluated a few years ago. Following an automobile accident in which she had sustained some neurological injury to her wrists, this woman failed to regain adequate function for a few years, even though the pressure on the nerves had been relieved. A neurologist employed by the defendant's insurance company had noted, "She tries to impress me how helpless she is. She asks my nurse to help her undress because the pain in her hands is too severe for her to do it by herself. She wears leather splints on both wrists and will not use her hands for anything. . . . She does not cooperate with the examination. She will not move her hands or extend her fingers. She makes absolutely no effort to grip with her hand. . . . All of this does indicate to me that she is malingering."

However, a psychiatrist concluded that she suffered from characteristics consistent with a somatization disorder or Briquet's disease. This is an illness in which the patient repeatedly focuses on real or imagined physical complaints. A careful review of her life history revealed that symptoms relating to a wide variety of organ systems had occurred since childhood. She had always been prone to pain and to fatigue, even when no monetary compensation was at issue. And there was a sort of bland underplaying, a degree of stoic martyrdom, in the way she reported her sickness—a characteristic often found in people with somatization disorder. For her to react with psychogenic pain, even after the tissue injuries cleared up, was certainly consistent with this diagnosis.

The diagnosis of malingering was further undercut when the psychiatrist repeated some of the neurologist's tests. Taking time to win her confidence, the psychiatrist got her to remove her wrist splints without help. Although she said that moving her fingers was painful, with encouragement, she moved them through a full range of motion. This examination occurred just one week before the trial. If she had been malingering, she needed to be "fully incapacitated" only seven more days. As a characterological trait, malingerers do not recover function just one week before trial. On the other hand, the symptoms of people with psychogenic pain wax and wane according to the situation. By analogy, removing a splinter hurts a child more in a climate of fear and brusqueness than in a climate of calm and gentleness.

The characterological approach may be helpful, but it is subject to pitfalls. Even inveterate liars may suffer mental illnesses. For example, criminal defendants with long and well-documented histories of schizophrenia may try rather ineptly to exaggerate their symptoms in an attempt to be even more convincing. Therefore, one can be both mentally ill and lying.

These guidelines used to detect malingering—consistency of the symptom pattern with a threshold mental illness and characterological behavior patterns—often are useful but not necessarily definitive. Psychiatrists can be fooled. It would be better if tests were available that did not depend on an inference that the patient is insincere or if there were tests of the threshold mental illness that did not depend on the patient's report.

Two tests used to support an inference of patient insincerity are the Minnesota Multiphasic Personality Inventory (MMPI) and the polygraph. The MMPI is a paper and pencil questionnaire that requires the person to indicate which statements describe him or her and which do not. Thus, although it is objective (i.e. anyone can score it and come up with the same results), it is also introspective (it requires the individual to report symptoms and mental attributes). Judges and juries sometimes confuse these two features and assume that because it is a TEST, the MMPI is not subject to insincerity. Actually, it is subject to the same falsification of reporting that may occur in a psychiatric interview, and the means by which this falsification may be detected are also the same. The MMPI is interpreted by examination of the patterns of responding, and there are certain patterns that are inconsistent with personality clusters and are consistent with the behavior of those people who attempt to deceive. And, as with the psychiatric interview and history, there is a sufficiently large number of people who fall in the grey area to make this test useful, but not definitive, (Graham, 1977, Chapters 3 and 8).

The polygraphy (lie detector), by contrast, does not depend on the internal consistency of symptoms reported. Instead, it measures physiological reactions, such as sweating, blood pressure, and breathing, while the patient is answering questions. These physiological functions vary with emotional excitement such as that generated when a patient feels he or she is being insincere. This method, then, would be a direct measure of lying that does not depend on the patient's reporting but on objective and extraspective data (data not based on the patient's inner mental life). Once again, judges and juries tend to put considerable reliance on the polygraph data because they have the trappings of science rather than intuition. The crucial link in the chain is whether these physiological measures do actually detect falsification. Podlesny and Raskin (1977) asserted that only 2 percent to 8 percent of those who are telling the truth give physiological measures indicating lying. However, Lykken (1979) maintained that this false positive range is actually 36 percent to 39 percent— clearly an unacceptable level. And, as Szucko and Kleinmutz (1981) have shown, the test is not really objective; the data must be interpreted by experienced judges, and there is considerable variability in their accuracy. In order to make the data analysis more objective, Szucko and Kleinmutz devised a statistical technique for analyzing polygraphic data, and while it proved more accurate than the interpretation by experienced judges, only "80% of the protocols could be classified correctly into their truthful and untruthful categories." And these data were obtained from the laboratory setting using psychology students who might be expected to have less general emotional variability than the gamut of people whose actions call for a *product of mental illness* decision.

So far, neither the psychiatric evaluation nor the tests to detect lying conclusively can rule out malingering in every case. Suppose, however, that doctors did not have to rely on the patient's report of symptoms. Suppose that there were directly observable physiological or anatomical indices of the threshold mental illnessess—

biological markers of disease. Then, there would be no need to depend on the sincerity of the person's report. Only if the biological markers were present, would the person have the threshold illness.

There are some biological indicators of certain mental illness. Intoxicants such as alcohol and drugs can be measured in the blood and urine. Tumors and other masses pressing on the brain may be detected by electroencephalography and various sophisticated X-ray techniques. Seizure disorders also often can be detected. Brain wave analysis of sleep patterns (Kupfer et al., 1978) and chemical tests of daily cycles of cortisol in the blood (Carroll et al., 1981) can be helpful in the diagnosis of depression. Recent studies using computerized integration of X ray data have raised the possibility of structural brain changes in schizophrenia (Andreasen et al., 1982), but these findings have been subject to question (Jernigan and Katz, 1981). Newer and even more sophisticated techniques using subatomic particles (positron emission tomography) and magnetic field studies (nuclear magnetic resonance) promise to give access to how much energy various parts of the brain are utilizing at any particular time. While the early studies are still equivocal, there is every reason to expect that biological markers will be developed for many of the threshold illnesses.

Will the development of valid biological markers of the threshold mental illnesses solve the malingering problems? Biological markers certainly could help define the threshold illness. Conceivably, some techniques such as positron emission tomography eventually might show energy modifications in specific areas of the brain that subserve certain specific functions, such as the capacity to understand or to delay urge. However, unless the crucial functions were altered all the time, (in which case there would be no need for the biological marker), the marker could not solve the allocation questions involved in *product* unless the biological measurements were taken at the time of the act. For example, suppose that certain biological indications of command hallucinations (voices instructing the patient to do certain acts) were available. Doctors know that psychotic people do not hallucinate all the time. Even if a biological marker of hallucinations were obtained at the time of testing, psychiatrists could not be certain that the individual was hallucinating at the time of the action in question. And even if doctors knew the patient was hallucinating during the action, they would not know what the voices were saying without relying on the individual's report. And even if it were possible to know to a certainty that the person heard a voice saying, "Kill" or "Sign the contract before it's too late," the fact remains that mentally ill people often hear commands that they resist. Biological markers will never solve the allocation problems in *product* decisions, even though they may eventually make psychiatrists more certain of the existence of the threshold mental illness. Most often doctors still will need to listen to the individual's explanations and decide if they are reasonably related to the act in question and are consistent with the kind of thinking found in the mental illness that has been diagnosed. These decisions still will depend to a significant degree on the policy decisions and emotional tugs described in Chapters Three and Four.

Thus, the problem of malingering remains. Who is to say that the person is insincere—the psychiatric expert or society's representatives? This question arose in the trial involving the auto accident victim who was unable to use her hands. The judge refused to admit the psychiatrist's testimony on the grounds that it was the jury's task to determine if the woman was telling the truth.

I do not entirely agree with this view. As experts, psychiatrists can state whether a cluster of reported mental characteristics has the internal consistency pointing to a mental illness. They can also comment on certain characterological features, especially as they bear on the psychological examination, as in the case of the woman who moved her hands one week before the trial.

When a cross-examining attorney challenges a professional psychiatrist by asking, "Doctor, have you ever been fooled?", he or she can reply, "Of course I have—probably more times than I am aware of. But here are the reasons why, in my opinion, I feel the plaintiff (or defendant) is not faking in this instance. . . . "

Other psychiatric experts may differ in their evaluation. Contradictory evidence may also be brought in by nonexpert witnesses. Ultimately, of course, it is the jury or some other representative designated by society that decides whom to believe or disbelieve, but the psychiatrist has some expertise in forming an opinion.

In certain situations, society may decide that some mental illnesses are too easily simulated and the issues involved are too important to run the risk of malingering. For example, in order to be brought to trial, a criminal defendant must be able to assist his or her attorney. Defendants will often claim amnesia for the offense and thus are unable to discuss the event with their lawyers. However, because amnesia is so easy to claim—"I just don't remember," and because it is so important for defendants to be brought to trial, amnesia has been excluded from the circle of threshold mental illnesses in the competency-to-stand-trial situations. In most situations, however, society has decided that the necessity for compassion for people with certain mental illnesses overrides the risk that these illnesses may be simulated. Society is not prepared to give up the *product of mental illness* questions merely because mental illness sometimes may be feigned. It is a less than perfect world, and to exclude all circumstances where lying is possible would deprive society of the compassion it requires as part of the emotional glue that holds it together.

CHAPTER SIX

OUTRAGE—COMPASSION
Criminal Responsibility

Probably no *product of mental illness* issue so stirs the emotions as does criminal responsibility. The question of *Sick or criminal?* taps the very deep springs of outrage and compassion. When an individual commits an offense, particularly against property or person, victims and onlookers alike become incensed. Personal safety and the security of the things counted as possessions are guaranteed only as long as the laws regulating society are upheld. Society respects order, and when this order is disrupted, people become upset, angry, and fearful.

Nonetheless, society recognizes that there may be mitigating circumstances in certain instances. Where the offense was an accident or was committed in self-defense, ordinarily the offender is not held responsible. At least as far back as the thirteenth century, unlawful action as a *product of mental illness* has been afforded the status of an exculpating circumstance (Amarillo, 1979). This is known as the insanity defense.

There is no basic logic which dictates that accident, self-defense, or mental illness should relieve the perpetrator of blame. If a person has been killed, he or she is just as dead regardless of the mental state of the killer. Money that has been taken and spent is gone, whether the taker meant to steal or suffered from a delusion that it was rightfully his or hers. At bottom, the blame is mitigated out of a sense of justice (*United States v Brawner*, 1972, Bazelon, J., partial dissent). Outrage is tempered with compassion by excusing the offender.

One indication of the strength of the emotional underpinnings of the insanity defense can be seen from the preeminence it has been given in political rhetoric. Mentally ill criminal defendants are the stuff of which newspaper sensationalism is made. Actually, a formal insanity defense is raised in only about 0.1 percent of criminal cases (Criss and Racine, 1980), and most of these do not result in acquittal. In Tennessee in 1977 to 1978, only twenty-four people out of over 500,000 criminal cases were found not guilty by reason of insanity (NGRI). And in most of these twenty-four cases, both the prosecuting and defense attorneys agreed that the defendant was seriously mentally ill. Thus, the insanity defense is the smallest part of the crime problem in the United States. Even if it were abolished entirely, there would be no appreciable effect on crime in this country. However, the issue captures the public's fancy and stirs their emotions, a fact that does not escape the notice of politicians who wish to appear hard on crime.

Now, although the insanity defense has captured the popular imagination, other procedures for resolving the *sick or criminal?* questions have gone virtually unnoticed despite the fact that they are employed far more frequently than is the insanity defense. In order to grasp this fact, one must have at least a rudimentary understanding of how an accused person is moved along the pathway of the judicial system. Either after direct observation or an investigation, the accused is taken into custody by a police officer. The policeman has considerable discretion to decide whether to take the person to a hospital or to jail (*sick or criminal?*). In Shelby County, Tennessee, over 2,000 people taken into custody annually are brought to the psychiatrists in the hospital emergency room for treatment rather than to the police station to be booked. Thus, over one hundred times as many offenders are declared sick rather than criminal by this informal procedure than by the more formal insanity defense.

After being taken by the officer to be booked, the accused goes through a complicated process wherein he or she may be charged with a crime, given an opportunity to plead guilty or innocent, try to work out a bargain with the prosecutor to plead guilty to a lesser charge, and raise certain legal issues. At these various points along the pathway to the trial, magistrates, judges, grand juries, and prosecutors may decide to treat the defendant as a sick person rather than as a criminal (Goldstein, 1967, Chapter 11). As we shall see in Chapter Ten, some of the decisions made along the pathway to the trial only appear to be *sick or criminal?* questions; even though they are phrased in that form, the real issues may be very different. Others, however, are bona fide *sick or criminal?* issues. Some of these decisions involve formal hearings while others merely are made informally.

The insanity defense comes into play only at the time of the trial, after all the preceding police, prosecutors, judges, magistrates, etc. have decided to treat the defendant as criminal rather than sick. The defendant, through his or her attorney, may then plead for a finding of not guilty on the ground that he or she was mentally ill at the time the offense occurred. It is at this point that the formal procedures and standards of insanity come into play. It is at this point that the relatively very few persons who are acquitted command the attention and emotions of the people, politicians, and the appellate courts.

Why does the insanity defense as a *sick or criminal?* decision that acquits comparatively few people arouse so much passion, while the earlier *sick or criminal?* decisions that acquit so many do not? Those whom the police bring to the hospital instead of to the police station are usually obviously ill. Often, their offense is not considered very serious because it arises in the context of home and family. There is little desire to prosecute. Compassion is high and outrage is minimal. Some of the same considerations are present when others in the pretrial procedures decide to drop the charges because of mental illness. This decision almost never is reached when the offense is serious or is one that offends the sensibilities of the community. Only cases where public outrage is low will be dropped. In other words, there is little public outcry about these *sick or criminal?* decisions because the public has little emotional stake in fixing blame. However, the cases that are not diverted to the mental health system before trial are the ones that provoke more outrage, and they may have little to recommend compassion. The cases where the insanity defense is invoked are battles fought on fields of high emotional pitch.

Since bona fide *sick or criminal?* decisions are not limited to the insanity defense, it may be useful to examine one other such decision process as well. In addition to the insanity defense, the police custody situation will be examined. In both situations, the dilemmas of the transductions and the expert role of the psychiatrist in the decision to label the deviant activity as a *product of mental illness* will be the focus of attention.

POLICE CUSTODY

COMPETING SOCIETAL INTERESTS. The purpose of having a police force goes far beyond that of apprehending criminals (Vanagunas and Elliot, 1980, pp. 19ff.). Among the many other functions are the preservation of peace and order, the protection of people and property, and the provision of a variety of emergency public services. In most jurisdictions, the police specifically are mandated by law to bring mentally ill people for help. When an officer is summoned to the scene of a disturbance, he or she can expect to perform any number of functions, only one of which is to apprehend a criminal. The whole gamut of deviant labels may lie before him or her: sick, criminal, unwise, merely unpleasant, or inexperienced, etc. Many factors, such as the seriousness of the disturbance, the wishes of the complainant, and the relationship between the deviant and those disturbed or harmed help determine whether the person will be taken into custody (Black, 1970). Once the decision has been made to apprehend the individual, there are essentially two dispositions—the mental illness route or the criminal justice route.

In the police custody situation, society does not send the officer in with the primary aim of declaring people criminal *unless* there is good reason for making exception. Rather, the officer serves several equally important societal interests. The police enter the scene of the disturbance equally prepared to express either outrage (criminal) or compassion (sick). In addition, only those cases where the offense is considered minor or relatively unimportant will be directed to the mental illness system. These situations evoke relatively little outrage, while the condition of the perpetrator arouses considerable compassion. Thus, there is not very much tension between the outrage and the compassion. If the disturbance evokes a high degree of outrage such as the case of a killing or rape, the perpetrator inevitably will be steered to the criminal justice system, with the question of mental illness to be decided at a later time.

By contrast, with the insanity defense, the individual already has been charged with a crime. The issue of criminality is highlighted, and society's interest in mental illness is primarily to carve out an exception. By the time of the trial, if the defendant pleads that the offense was a *product of mental illness*, a high level of outrage has developed and the question is whether there will be sufficient compassion to overcome it. In this situation, both emotions may run high thus increasing the tension between them.

The specific interests society has in capturing criminals will be reviewed in more detail later in the discussion of the insanity defense. Society's purposes in taking mentally ill people into custody will be discussed in the following chapter when commitment issues are considered. It is sufficient to note at this point that there are long-established rationales for each of these courses — treating deviant and disruptive people as criminals or as mentally ill persons. These rationales rest on outrage when the criminal path is chosen and on compassion when the officer chooses the mental illness course.

STANDARDS. While society has set certain standards for determining whether a mentally ill person should be taken into custody (see Chapter Seven), the officer is given no formal standards to help him or her distinguish between mentally ill people and criminals. In this *sick or criminal?* situation, there are no criteria of sufficient mental illness. Given a situation where the person must be apprehended, usually because of serious disturbance or danger, the officer is left to his or her own devices to determine whether to take the individual to the hospital or to the police station.

What standards are available are informal. As a matter of police practice, if the offense is not considered to be very serious, the disruptive person is treated as sick if the question of suicide is raised, if the behavior in question is incongruous and not easily understood, or if the person is disoriented (Bitner, 1967).

There are two ways in which the psychiatrist plays a role in setting up these informal standards. Either by writing police training manuals or by direct participation as a lecturer in the training academy, the psychiatrist teaches the police recruit how to recognize mental illness. In doing this, the psychiatrist is subtly making a transduction. Even if the information is couched in the strictest terms of diagnostic criteria, the message to the recruits is clear: Of all the people who cause disturbances, these are the ones who likely are not to be able to control themselves. As pointed out earlier in this book, this implication goes well beyond psychiatric expertise. There is no way around this problem when psychiatrists give such training other than to make very certain to emphasize that these people, while sick, may have also committed a crime, and that the decision about which route to take must be up to the officer. While the police use this training, they have wide discretion to use their own judgement and set their own standards. In essence, this is a two-transduction procedure for setting standards.

The second way the psychiatrist participates in setting the informal standards is even more subtle. After the individual has been taken to the hospital, it is the psychiatrist who decides whether admission is needed. At this juncture, the psychiatrist may apply the formal criteria for involuntary hospitalization (see Chapter Seven). If the patient is not admitted, the officer, after having invested considerable time and energy, is still left with an "aggravated problem on his hands" (Bitner, 1967). The police quickly learn which types of individuals are likely to be accepted as sick by the hospitals and which are likely to be rejected. In subsequent cases, those who are likely to be rejected may be diverted to the criminal pathway.

The police officer's decision between sick or criminal, of course, is not final; it is subject to review by a more formal system. If the person is taken to the police station, the decision to declare that he or she is a criminal may be modified in subsequent procedings. If the person is taken to the hospital, the decision to declare him or her as sick is subject to review by the doctor. Therefore, it may make sense not to define too rigorously a circle of conditions that will weed out the sick from the criminal at this stage. The present informal system of standards gives the police a maximum of flexibility to apply the "robust common sense" of the society of which they are representatives.

DECIDING THE INDIVIDUAL CASE. There are many factors that help determine whether the police will treat a disruptive person as sick or criminal. The situation at the scene of the disturbance and the ease of getting people admitted to the hospital will both affect the decision. However, when the initial *sick or criminal?* decision is made at the scene of the disturbance, no psychiatrist is involved and there are no problems of opinion masquerading as professional expertise. The officer weighs the facts and decides whether this particular individual fits the informal standards of people who society feels are unable to control themselves.

Once the individual has been brought to the hospital, however, the psychiatrist does become a participant. Optimally, the psychiatrist should not become involved in the *sick or criminal?* question at this point. The individual should be evaluated on the same basis as any other prospective patient. If he or she meets the criteria for hospitalization (see Chapter Seven), the person should be admitted. If treatment is indicated but hospitalization is not warranted, the individual should be treated and returned to the custody of the officer. Generally, treatment in this setting consists of two types. The agitated individual may be medicated and referred for follow-up outpatient treatment while the person not requiring medication will be talked to, calmed down if necessary, and referred for follow-up outpatient treatment if it seems indicated. In either situation, the well-functioning emergency room (of which there are all too few) will also work with family members to help cool down the situation. When the treated person is returned to the custody of the police, the implication is that he or she is no longer likely to be dangerous (the person would have been hospitalized otherwise). At this point, the officer can decide to release the individual (sick but improved), or if the disturbance aroused sufficient outrage, the person can be charged with a crime.

For example, a twenty-three-year-old man was brought to the emergency room because he was threatening suicide. He had had a stormy on-again, off-again relationship with his girlfriend who had become increasingly upset by his physical abuse of her when he drank. On this occasion, while drunk, he hit her sufficiently hard to leave bruises. When she threatened to break up with him "once and for all," he said that he would kill himself if she left. This alarmed her, and she called the police. While she was angry because of the beating, the woman was also concerned about her boyfriend's potential for suicide. The officer could have treated this case as assault and battery (criminal), but he decided that the suicide threat made the man more sick than criminal. The girlfriend agreed.

After talking with the man, psychiatrists ascertained that he was feeling very sorry for himself, but he had never entertained seriously the intention of killing himself; the threat was used as a means of regaining his girl friend. He was referred for the treatment of his alcoholism and the woman was encouraged to seek the assistance of a spouse-abuse group.

It was not the responsibility of psychiatrists to persuade either the woman or the officer to press charges for the abuse, no matter how incensed the professionals might have been at the man's behavior. For the psychiatrist to say to the officer that the man is not sick, but rather he is manipulating in order to get out of the criminal charge, etc., implies knowledge that he could have acted differently if he wanted to—a conclusion that goes beyond expertise, as explained in Chapters Two and Three. If appropriate, the woman and the officer can be informed of the results of the interview with the boyfriend, and they should be told that he is not suicidal. But it is up to them and their outrage and compassion to decide if he is the kind of person whom they feel could not control his behavior (sick) or if he was mean and wily (criminal). It is the officer who must decide to release him (sick, but no longer dangerous) or book him (criminal).

Sometimes no treatment seems indicated, either because the individual does not want it or because the person has a condition for which there is no treatment. In this situation, unless the person meets the requirements for involuntary hospitalization (Chapter Seven), the psychiatrist should return the person to the police officer for disposition. For example, for several years, a middle-aged woman had accused a city official of having raped her many years previously. She said that one of his children was hers rather than his wife's. She had never taken him to court, nor had she ever made an attempt to gain custody of the child. Indeed, she never even tried to talk with the youngster. Instead, from time to time, she would parade in front of his house telling passersby about the terrible injustice the official was inflicting on her.

The woman had been hospitalized involuntarily on several occasions and all the psychiatrists who examined her agreed that the diagnosis of paranoid disorder was appropriate. Although she had received several types of medication, as is so often the case with this condition, her delusion was unshakable. The condition followed its own course. At times it was not pronounced and although she still felt she had lost her child, she made no fuss about it; while at other times it was more prominent and she resumed her protest in front of the official's house. He, of course, was very upset, and he wanted her removed. However, she was so obviously sick, he was reluctant to have her arrested.

One night she was again brought to the emergency room. The psychiatrist who evaluated her reached the same conclusion as had his predecessors. She was suffering from a paranoid disorder; no effective treatment was available, and since she was not dangerous, she could not be hospitalized involuntarily. He gave this information to the police and returned the woman to their custody. At that point, it was up to them to decide whether to label her behavior sick and release her, unpleasant and release her, or criminal and arrest her if they could work out appropriate charges.

If the psychiatrist remembers the limits of the expert role and resists the temptation to use his or her position to dictate public morality, it should be possible to refrain from making *sick or criminal?* decisions in the police custody situation. This is not always easy to do, especially in a busy emergency room. Not infrequently, overworked psychiatrists become angry with the flood of prospective patients and tend to view more and more of them as manipulators who are using illness to avoid being held responsible for their actions. However, professionals must remember that people may manipulate as a part or in reaction to mental illness (Bursten, 1973a). The manipulation is usually irrelevant to the psychiatrist's task in the police custody situation unless it consists of malingering. If the illness is feigned (see Chapter Five), there is nothing to treat, and the police should be so informed. However, if the condition is not feigned but is a diagnosis that the psychiatrist does not wish to be burdened with—usually alcohol or drug related or personality disorders—the individual should be referred elsewhere, or, when appropriate, told that there is no treatment available. It is not the psychiatrist's role to tell the police that the person is not sick because there are no formal standards for sufficient mental illness in the police custody situation. Nor is it the expert role of the psychiatrist to say that the individual is trying to escape criminal activity. That decision, that transduction, should be reserved for the police.

INSANITY DEFENSE

COMPETING SOCIETAL INTERESTS. The insanity defense situation differs from the police custody situation in several ways. This *sick or criminal?* decision takes place at the time of the trial. The individual in question is now a defendant accused of a crime. There is usually a fair amount of evidence indicating that he or she perpetrated the act; otherwise the prosecutor would not have carried the case this far. The offense is serious enough to warrant the time and expense of prosecution, and if it is that serious, it is capable of evoking considerable outrage from the public and their representatives who will make the decision — the jury. In order for the insanity defense to prevail, the jury must have sufficient compassion for the defendant to temper its outrage. The emotions and the tension between them are high.

The trial, if it is conducted correctly, is the final decision point. It is more definitive than the police custody situation. Since society has a very high stake in seeing that it is fair, it is subject to considerable public and judicial scrutiny. Therefore, the rules by which the decision is made are much more formal, and there is an attempt to reduce the discretion of the decisionmakers.

Since society's emotional pitch is high in the insanity defense situation and the decision process is much more formalized than in the case of the police custody *sick or criminal?* situation, a more detailed examination will be presented concerning the strong competing interests that society has in convicting defendants if they are criminal and exculpating them if they are sick.

Goldstein (1967, p. 15) has pointed out that " ... underlying all [themes in the criminal law], as the single constant element, is the concept of blame." If an offense has been committed, society wants to hold someone responsible. The purposes of fixing blame are made clearer by the consequences of being found guilty: fines, imprisonment or probation (the threat of imprisonment), or sometimes death. According to Hart (1958), these consequences may have a rehabilitative function, act as a deterrent to others, protect the rest of society by segregating bad people, sharpen the community's sense of right and wrong, promote the concept that each individual is responsible for making society work, and satisfy society's need for vengeance and retribution. Each of these aims directs attention to a legitimate societal interest in finding offenders blameworthy and guilty. To some degree, they all reflect society's outrage (with its fear component); however, vengeance and retribution speak loudest about outrage while segregation speaks most directly to fear.

On the other hand, society also has a compassionate interest in exempting mentally ill people from criminal responsibility. In the first place, the law has long held that basic to blame and guilt is the concept of *mens rea*. This was defined by Perkins (1939) as a state of mind "sufficient for criminal guilt" and by the Supreme Court (*United States v Freed,* 1971) as "vicious will." In other words, it is not sufficient to perpetrate the act; to be held criminally responsible one must simultaneously be in a morally bad frame of mind. This does not necessarily mean that the accused must have intended to do the act; he or she may have been reckless and disregarded the possible consequences of the action, or he or she was negligent and failed to take the precautions everyone is expected to take. This principle allows society to have compassion for those offenders whom are felt not to be in a morally bad frame of mind. For example, if a man with paranoid schizophrenia killed his parents because he believed them to be imposters placed at his home by some foreign conspiracy in order to overthrow the government and to be in a position to burn the 135 children he has fathered, it may be decided that he lacked mens rea and society's temper may be outraged with compassion.

In the second place, the Eighth Amendment prohibits cruel and unusual punishment. According to Grannucci (1969), this concept arose in England during the seventeenth century because punishments were being administered that were disproportionate to the offenses. In 1931, a Mississippi court stated that to convict a person who was insane at the time of the offense would be cruel and unusual punishment (*Sinclair u State*, 1931). As Chief Justice Warren said, "[The Eighth Amendment] must draw its meaning from the evolving standards of decency that mark the progress of a maturing society" (*Trop u Dulles*, 1958). The Eighth Amendment then, acts as a compassionate brake on the unbridled expression of outrage toward the offender.

A third societal interest, oddly enough, is expressed by the view that excusing mentally ill people from criminal responsibility actually makes the concept of guilt and personal responsibility more tenable. Packer (1968, pp. 132ff.) noted that in order to support the "robust common sense" assumption of free will, society must recognize "that some people are, by reason of mental illness, significantly impaired in their volitional capacity." If humans are endowed with volition, it can be impaired. And Stone (1976, p. 222) said, "But what is a court to do when it confronts a case so bizarre and so incongruous that all the premises of criminal law, including free will, seem inappropriate? ... The insanity defense is in every. sense the exception that proves the rule. It allows the court to treat every other defendant as someone who chooses 'between good and evil.'" It seems that what these writers are expressing in intellectual terms is the very human need to temper outrage with compassion in certain instances.

A fourth societal interest is that of rehabilitation. Theoretically, at least, one might argue that a defendant who could have controlled his or her actions might learn a lesson by going to prison. However, since a person whose offense was a *product of mental illness* could not control him or herself, no learning can take place; rehabilitation is best achieved by treating the illness that caused the offense.

Now, although the insanity defense serves as a method of tempering outrage with compassion, it does not fully overcome the outrage. Goldstein and Katz (1963) noted that the consequence of a successful insanity plea was incarceration, albeit in a mental hospital rather than in a jail. They implied that the compassionate thrust was somewhat of a sham—a device to provide a way of segregating those offenders who, because they lacked mens rea, could not be jailed. This view is supported by the public outcry when an individual, acquitted by reason of insanity, is released from the mental hospital after only a short period of time. Rather than rejoicing that the person has so quickly been relieved of his or her mental illness (compassion), the public feels that the person has been insufficiently punished for the offense (outrage).

However, the process is not quite a sham. It is not a situation of *either* outrage *or* compassion, but rather a tension between the two emotions that may sometimes tilt more toward one emotion and sometimes tilt more toward the other. Society does have compassion for the legally insane defendant, but not so much compassion that it wants to see him or her go free. This would be "too upsetting . . . some incubation period is necessary to allow time for public outrage to be dissipated . . . " (Goldstein, 1967, p. 145). On the other hand, society does not have so little compassion that it is willing to treat every offender in the same fashion regardless of his or her mental state. Thus, a review of the whole process, it can be demonstrated that keeping the legally insane defendant out of jail does reflect real compassion. Only when the individual is kept in the hospital over a long period of time does the compassion become a sham—outrage masquerading as compassion. This situation will be further considered in Chapter Ten.

When society's policymakers attempt to balance these competing interests in order to forge procedures and standards for the insanity defense, they are strongly influenced by the temper of the times. The procedures (which were mentioned in Chapter Four) and the standards are shaped so that greater or fewer numbers of defendants can be found not guilty by reason of insanity when society shifts back and forth between more outrage and more compassion. As various standards are examined, it will be shown how the policy makers have been responsive to these shifts.

STANDARDS. Since the insanity defense has been around since the thirteenth century, it is not surprising that the standards have undergone many changes. In the Middle Ages, rough cognitive tests such as the ability to count or to recognize one's parents were used to differentiate the legally sane from the legally insane (Amarillo, 1979). In the sixteenth century, England adopted a set of rules for determining legal insanity, which were dependent on a knowledge of good and evil and were substantially like the later

M'Naughten Rule. However, in 1800, the standard was broadened to encompass all acts that resulted from mental illness (*United States u Currens,* 1961). Some of the more recent standards that have been used since that time will be examined.

The M'Naughten Rule.

Slovenko (1973, p. 78) has described the emotional wave that swept *M'Naughten* into existence. Daniel M'Naughten felt persecuted by the Torries who were in power in England in the mid 1800s. He decided to take action against them by killing Sir Robert Peel, the prime minister. He kept a watch on Peel's house, and when he saw a man emerge, he shot him. It was a mistake, however; the victim was not Peel but Edward Drummond. At the trial, the jury found M'Naughten not guilty on the grounds of insanity. The acquittal was the beginning rather than the end of that celebrated drama.

> Although acquitted of crime, M'Naughten was certified as being of unsound mind and detained in a lunatic asylum where he spent his remaining 22 years. The verdict of not guilty on the grounds of insanity, however, created a furor, and within a few days after the trial the case was debated in the House of Lords. It was speculated that M'Naughten, a Scotsman, was a political assassin. The times were turbulent. Shortly before, Queen Victoria had been the target of an assassination attempt by an assailant who was also found not guilty by reason of insanity. On learning of the M'Naughten acquittal, she summoned the House of Lords to an extraordinary session. They were instructed to clarify and tighten the concept of criminal responsibility. They came forth with the so-called M'Naughten rules. . . .

which were, in fact, a replay of rules outlined three centuries earlier.

The M'Naughten Rules state that to qualify as legally insane, "the accused must have had such a defect of reason, from disease of the mind, as not to know the nature and quality of the act he was doing; or if he did know it, that he did not know he was doing what was wrong" (*M'Naughten's Case,* 1843). This standard requires someone to state if a defendant had a mental illness, if he or she had more specific defects in the cognitive sphere, and if there were a causal relationship between them and the act in question. It poses the typical *product* dilemmas of defining who is mentally ill and allocating the behavior between the sick and healthy parts of the person. It should be noted that even if cognitive defects can be identified, such as delusional thinking, the question of whether the individual's choosing mechanism was crippled by this sick function or whether it was intact and responding to coexisting healthy contexts of the situation still must be confronted.

The Irresistible Impulse Rule

According to Guttmacher (1968), "The concept of loss of control, without a corresponding disturbance of cognition, was recognized in French law early in the nineteenth century. It appears to have been recognized in England in 1840 (when a jury was instructed) that if some controlling disease was, in truth, the acting power within him which he could not resist 'they were to bring in a verdict of insanity.' " This standard and its implications are stated most clearly in *Parsons v State* (1887). If "by reason of the duress of (a) mental disease, (the defendant) has so far lost the *power* to choose between right and wrong, and to avoid doing the act in question, as that his free agency was at the time destroyed . . . and if, at the same time, the alleged crime was so connected with the mental disease, in the relation of cause and effect, as to have been the product of it solely," an insanity verdict is to be rendered. Once again, the decisionmaker must determine if the individual in question has a mental illness—this time affecting the urge rather than the cognitive functions. And psychiatrists must still allocate the action between the sick and healthy parts to determine if the choosing mechanism was overridden.

The Durham Rule

By the mid 1950s, fifteen states, the federal jurisdictions, and the United States Army had expanded the M'Naughten Rule by adding to it the Irresistible Impulse Rule (American Law Institute, 1955). This was a period of therapeutic optimism. Sparked by psychoanalytic observations, the intellectual community tilted toward the deterministic framework, and hitherto inexplicable behavior that had been ascribed to moral badness was now understood in terms of subtle causes rooted in brain and mental processes (Alexander and Staub, 1956). Following the standard in use in New Hampshire since 1870, the D.C. Circuit court promulgated the "simple" rule that "an accused is not criminally responsible if his unlawful act was the product of mental disease or defect" (*Durham v. U.S.*, 1954). In essence, the court had returned the District of Columbia to where England had been before M'Naughten.

While many psychiatrists saw the Durham decision as allowing the jury to make use of the latest advances in psychiatry (Slovenko, 1973, p. 80), the lawyers were of a more practical bent. According to Arens (1974, p. 2), "practicing lawyers in the District of Columbia saw the rule almost intuitively as inviting *compassion* as well as a more careful and comprehensive scientific assessment. . . . " (italics mine).

Of course, by definition, the *Durham* standard suffered from all the problems of every *product* standard. In addition, because it did not even give the appearance of standards, it exposed the basic dilemmas of both *mental illness* and *product* (*Blocker v. United States* 1961, Burger, J., concurring the result only).

The American Law Institute (ALI) Test.

This standard, formulated by the ALI (1962) is as follows:

> (1) A person is not responsible for criminal conduct if at the time of such conduct, as a result of mental disease or defect, he lacks substantial capacity either to appreciate the criminality (wrongfulness) of his conduct or to conform his conduct to the requirements of the law;
>
> (2) As used in this article, the terms 'mental disease or defect' do not include an abnormality manifested only by repeated criminal or otherwise antisocial conduct.

The *product* dilemmas are found in the first paragraph, which are a combination of the cognitive M'Naughten Rule, the urge Irresistible Impulse Rule, plus the provision for conduct caused by intense emotions.

Diminished Capacity.

In the 1980s, public outrage is again on the rise. Society has become alarmed by an ever-increasing crime rate and the fact that a defendant such as John Hinckley, who attempted to assassinate President Reagan, was found not guilty by reason of insanity. The public and the politicians are in no mood to have much compassion for serious offenders.

One proposal, adopted by Idaho, has been to abolish the insanity defense but to allow testimony relevant to diminished capacity (Carnahan et al., 1978; I.C., sections 18–205, 207, 1981). Diminished capacity is used to temper outrage with compassion by reducing the seriousness of the crime (and hence the prison sentence) while not acquitting the defendant altogether. It is based on the proposition that certain crimes require specific mental states. For example, first degree murder often requires that the defendant premeditate (plan the killing) and be able to deliberate (reflect on the action and its possible consequences). Second degree murder, which carries a lighter sentence, does not require these capacities; even if there is no premeditation or deliberation, however, the individual must be able to appreciate that his or her actions run a high likelihood that someone would be killed.

While this standard makes no provision for acquittal and therefore tilts heavily toward outrage, the *product* dilemmas, which are the focus of this book, remain. Society still inquires about the defendant's "mental condition and symptoms, his pathological beliefs and motives" and "how these influence or could have influenced his behavior" (*Rhodes v United States*, 1960). In one of the classic diminished capacity cases (*People v Gorshen*, 1959), Diamond testified that the "medical essence of malice aforethought" (a mental state necessary to raise the seriousness of the crime) was the question of whether the defendant acted out of free will or because of an abnormal force or compulsion.

American Psychiatric Association (APA) Proposal.

Swept along by the public furor about recent insanity defense trials, the APA, for the first time in its 138 year history, issued a statement on the insanity defense standards (APA News, February 4, 1983). The defendant should be declared legally insane if he or she were "unable to appreciate the wrongfulness of the conduct at the time of the offense" that resulted from a "severly abnormal mental condition." This condition, "usually a psychosis," must impair the defendant's "perception or understanding of reality." Conditions such as alcohol and drug intoxication and personality disorders such as antisocial personality disorders should not qualify.

This proposal, unlike the preceding ones, attempts to delineate threshold mental illnesses, although by using the phrase "usually a psychosis," it becomes a bit ambiguous. There is still considerable room for debate about whether conditions that are neither specifically included nor excluded, such as dissociative disorder, nonantisocial personality disorders, or intermittent explosive disorder, are to be considered as "severely abnormal mental conditions." Nonetheless, it is a step toward the concept of sufficient mental illness as suggested in Chapter Four.

The proposal also attempts to revert to the M'Naughten (cognitive) standard. Because the ability to control behavior "is a subject of some disagreement among psychiatrists," emotion and urge functions are disallowed. However, the *product* relationship, along with the necessity for a transduction at the decision-making stage, is implied, if not specifically stated. It is not the determination that the defendant could not appreciate the wrongfulness of the act which is crucial; what is important is the conclusion that the behavior was performed because of this lack of appreciation and would not have been done if there had been better appreciation.

As the history of the insanity defense is reviewed the disappearance and subsequent reappearance of various standards is seen in response to many factors, not the least of which is the temper of the times. It is difficult to know if changing the standards actually has the effect of increasing or reducing the number of people acquitted by reason of insanity (Simon, 1967; Arens, 1974). Juries, like policymakers, may alter the balance of outrage — compassion in response to the emotional climate of society, and changes in the statistics may reflect this effect rather than the results of changing the standards.

However, when examining the history of the various standards, one thing becomes clear: Any standard inevitably will lead to dissatisfaction. The reasons for this are that the insanity defense has high social visibility (in contrast, for example, to the police custody decision), society goes through swings of greater or lesser outrage towards crime, and the experts—psychiatrists—so easily are exposed as making policy rather than scientific decisions. Any standard that depends on mental illness requires the expert to perform a transduction from determinism to libertarianism. Adding specific mental characteristics such as limiting the standards to the cognitive sphere will not help, because any skillful rhetorician— lawyer or doctor—will make a mockery of the limitation as Goldstein (1967, Chapter 4) has suggested. Longer and more wordy explanations to help define the precise mental state within the circle do not really resolve the problem; one cannot solve this transduction problem by throwing words at it. Unless a concept of sufficient mental illness together with threshold diagnoses is incorporated into the standards, an unsolvable dilemma remains.

While the APA proposal moves in the direction of setting up threshold mental conditions, the framers have gone beyond their area of expertise in doing so. There is no psychiatric wisdom which dictates that, for example, people with antisocial personalities should be excluded from the circle of allowable illnesses, although there may be some political wisdom in taking this course. ·Which types of people are those whom society expects should be able to conform is a matter for society's policymakers. The members of the APA committee have made their own transduction; as psychiatrists, they have used their knowledge of various mental conditions to activate themselves as citizens expressing "robust common sense" based on the tension between outrage and compassion. This should at least be made explicit to the policymakers.

DECIDING THE INDIVIDUAL CASE. Despite what the psychiatrist says in testimony, it is the jury that ultimately decides whether to grant the defendant the status of not guilty by reason of insanity (*Washington v. United States*, 1967). These twelve representatives of society have the final say about whether the defendant is the kind of person whom society feels could have behaved better if he or she wanted to. However, there is some evidence that they may follow the lead of the psychiatrist, especially if the examination has been done under the auspices of the court rather than for the defense. And, even more relevant to the argument of this book is the suggestive evidence that those psychiatrists who are on the neutral court examining teams are influenced in their decisions by the same outrage and compassion swings that affect society at large (Steadman et al., 1983).

Theoretically, it is the job of the decision maker to see if the defendant fits the standard. Since it is the jury that is the decision maker, it would be appropriate to confine the psychiatrists to the presentation of facts and medical (as contrasted with social) opinions. However, this is impossible when the standard is "mental illness." It is also impossible when the standard is "severe mental illness." Does a narcissistic person who flies into a rage when frustrated have a severe mental abnormality (Bursten, 1981)? Does not "severe" really mean "severe enough to count"? Inserting the word *severe* makes the issue no more factual than did the word *substantial,* which was inserted twenty years earlier (*McDonald v. United States,* 1962).

As discussed in Chapter Four, unless the specific threshold diagnoses have been spelled out, the psychiatrist-witness must leave the sphere of his or her expertise. And even if the standards were to specify certain diagnostic categories, if the psychiatrist must testify whether the behavior resulted from any particular illness, a transduction must be made. The APA proposed a standard which requires that the ability to appreciate the wrongfulness can be impaired. The bottom line is whether the choosing mechanism has been more affected by the impairment or by the healthy parts of the person — allocation.

The only way to ensure that this dilemma is avoided is to use the one-transduction system outlined in Chapter Four. Essentially, in this procedure, the standards would specify specific threshold illnesses and the psychiatrist would testify about them. If specific mental characteristics were included, the psychiatrist could comment about them also. But the healthy parts would also be presented, and the psychiatrist would make no conclusions about which parts (sick or healthy) were dominant. This conclusion, this transduction, would be left to the jury.

There is no certainty that such a system is feasible or practical. However, without it, a two-transduction system exists, and no matter how it is twisted or turned, society always will be confronted with the dilemma of the psychiatric testimony going beyond professional expertise. Psychiatrists should tell the jury what they are doing and stop worrying about it.

CHAPTER SEVEN

COMPASSION—INDIFFERENCE

The Right to be Left Alone

In recent years, much of the litigation involving psychiatric practice has been carried forth by attorneys interested in civil liberties. Writers from Szasz (1963) to Robitscher (1980) have warned the public that psychiatrists, acting on their own or as agents of the government, may be riding roughshod over the rights of individuals designated as sick.

The basic right that has concerned these commentators is the right to be left alone, to be free from government intervention. It has been called "the most comprehensive of rights and the right most valued by civilized men" (*Olmstead v United States*, 1928, Brandeis, J. dissenting). It stands out as a fundamental political value in America, a bulwark against governmental oppression. Government and its agents may abridge individual liberties only when there are compelling justifications. And where there is justification, any deprivation of liberty must be done under legal safeguards.

One must be very careful about the use of the words *freedom* and *liberty*, because they are sufficiently ambiguous to be used in rhetorical advantage. The liberty referred to in this book is an immune right—freedom from government intervention. Advocates of compulsory treatment will often argue that they, too, are for freedom—the right of the individual to be free from the crippling effects of illness. This is not an immune right; it is a claim and thus is a very different (even if important) type of freedom. Essentially, it is a claim that everyone is entitled to health and that the state has an obligation to provide it. This claim will be discussed in Chapter Eight. In terms of the focus of the present book, the individual who is exercising his or her immune right says, "I'm not sick, let me be on my own"; the person exercising a claim says, "I am sick, don't leave me on my own."

In a variety of situations, society feels that, because the individual in question is mentally ill, the right to be left alone should be abridged. In general, abridgement of this right is justified on the grounds that the person is not really competent to make a sound decision. Society, in its compassion, wishes to step in to prevent the person from embarking on a foolish course while the individual wishes to be treated with indifference. This is usually a *sick or unwise?* question. Is the behavior under scrutiny a *product of mental illness* or merely the result of a poorly thought out plan and a bad decision? Among the many types of *sick or unwise?* situations involving the right to be left alone, five examples will be considered: the decision to refuse mental hospitalization, hospitalization of political dissenters, the decision to refuse treatment in the mental hospital, the decision to refuse treatment for nonmental illnesses, and the desire of the elderly to manage their own affairs. By way of contrast, the decision to have rhinoplasty also will be considered.

In all of these situations as considered in this chapter, the fulcrum of the balance of compassion and indifference is the issue of whether the individual in question is competent to make his or her own decision. Therefore, this issue should be examined briefly before proceeding to the specific situations.

While the question of incompetence touches on a wide variety of "right to be left alone" issues, surprisingly little attention has been devoted to problems of the standards by which an individual can be judged incompetent. At the base of the standard, of course, is the requirement that the person be mentally ill; however, there is no incompetence standard that specifies just which mental illnesses count and which do not. In every case, the transduction necessary to define the mental illness that qualifies for incompetence is left to the decision maker.

In addition to the requirement of mental illness, virtually all tests of incompetence require certain specific, cognitive features of that illness. The general rule is that the individual be unable to appreciate the nature or possible consequences of the decision in question or to understand his or her relationship to the decision. The person who grasps what the decision is all about in the abstract but cannot grasp that he or she is the one involved would be incompetent.

Roth et al. (1977) have attempted to spell out in somewhat greater detail the cognitive functions as they may be used as tests of incompetence. A person who, as a feature of mental illness, fails to state a preference (e.g. a mute, catatonic, schizophrenic person) is usually considered incompetent. Other cognitive tests may include electing a course that has an unreasonable outcome (one that a reasonable person would not make), deciding on the basis of irrational reasons, or evidencing, as a feature of the mental illness, a persistent lack in the understanding of the decision situation. This lack of understanding may result from two circumstances: In the first place, the person may not have been given enough information; this would be lack of informed consent, not incompetence. In the second place, the person may have been adequately informed, but because of the mental illness, is unable to assimilate the information; this is incompetence. Thus, in any examination, the first step is to ascertain if the person understands; if actual understanding is lacking, the reason for the lack must be sought.

In addition to the cognitive tests, some tests of incompetence use a broader standard. They may designate mental functions in the emotive and urge spheres, and in this manner they enlarge the circle of people judged incompetent.

All of these cognitive, emotive, and urge functions and the decisions that are based on them must be products of the acceptable mental illness in order for incompetence to be declared. And regardless of the specific mental functions specified, regardless of how many words thrown into the definitions, the decisionmaker must allocate *product* by making a transduction. Thus, in every situation where the right to be left alone is abridged by a judgement of incompetence, the same basic *product* dilemmas are encountered that are woven into the issues of criminal responsibility described in the previous chapter.

REFUSING MENTAL HOSPITALIZATION

COMPETING SOCIETAL INTERESTS. As late as 1969, a state court (*Prochaska v. Brinegar*, 1960) held that the right to refuse mental hospitalization is not the sort of liberty protected by Constitutional guarantees. By the 1970s, however, federal courts were calling commitment "a massive curtailment of liberty" (*Humphrey v. Cady*, 1972), and they placed involuntary hospitalization under the protective cloak of the Fourteenth Amendment (*In re Ballay*, 1973).

In addition to the strong Constitutional interest in protecting people from forced hospitalization, there are other arguments supporting the prospective patient's right to be left alone. Dix (1981) has cited the unpleasantness of hospitalization as well as the loss of privacy and sense of autonomy. Then, too, there is a stigma attached to commitment. One joins the class of "ex-mental patients" who may be excluded from certain occupations, from owning a gun, and sometimes, at least temporarily, from the right to drive a car. As an "exmental patient," one's social situation is often different from that of other people.

Counterbalancing these factors are society's interests in abridging the right to refuse hospitalization. Two concepts are invoked to justify this abridgment—police power and parens patriae (Livermore et al., 1968; Kittrie, 1971, Chapter 1; Developments in the Law, 1974). Police power is the power of the State to make laws and regulations protecting the public health, safety, welfare, and morals. From the standpoint of the commitment issue, police power will refer to the maintenance of public safety. Parens patriae is the power the State assumes in order to care for those unfortunate citizens who cannot care for themselves.

Police power has been around as long as there have been governments. When a person is considered potentially dangerous to people or property, society is no longer willing to treat him or her with indifference; outrage with its fear component is stirred and police power justifications are mobilized. Since the individual may not have commited a serious crime, since he or she is merely likely (in the future) to do significant harm, the criminal justice system cannot be utilized. However, society can protect itself by placing the person in a mental hospital. Now there is a problem here. Not everyone who appears imminently dangerous or seems likely to threaten the public's safety is hospitalized. What about the person with a bad temper? What about the political activist whose rhetoric causes others to fear violence? What about vehemently argumentative people, people who get into barroom brawls or people who hate others? The *mentally ill and* dangerous are singled out for involuntary hospitalization. People whose apparent dangerousness results from mental illness are separated from others because society feels that they cannot control themselves, while it is felt that other potentially violent people could control themselves if they so desired. There are two ways to interpret this justification of involuntary hospitalization. In the first view, society may decide it is necessary to segregate out-of-control people who are apparently dangerous regardless of whether they are competent or incompetent to make their own decisions (*Rogers v Okin,* 1980). This is more of an outrage— indifference situation than a case of compassion—indifference; society is not concerned primarily about the welfare of the individual in question. This situation will be considered in Chapter Ten.

In the second view, not only the public but also the individual in question is being protected from the consequences of his or her actions (Developments in the Law, 1974). This out-of-control person must be kept out of trouble; he or she is viewed more compassionately. But what if the person does not want to be treated so compassionately? What if he or she wants to be left alone to take his or her chances like the other dangerous people? Then the incompetence standard is invoked; society deprives the individual of the right to make that decision on the grounds that the refusal of hospitalization is a *product of mental illness.* Underneath the outrage toward the dangerous person lies the compassion for the sick individual whose choosing mechanism is crippled. It is this view of the dangerousness criterion that will be discussed in the present chapter.

As such, there are two aspects to the criteria of commitment: The first stage involves the social aspect—dangerousness to others. This is the threshold aspect that triggers society's interest and leads to the offer of hospitalization. When the individual refuses that offer, the second aspect—incompetence to decide whether hospitalization is needed—is invoked.

There are a variety of social aspect criteria. While dangerousness to others is a police power justification, parens patriae justifications such as dangerousness to oneself or merely the need for care and treatment are also employed. Parens patriae (father of the country) indicates that the king (or State) has parental responsibility for the citizens. According to Kittrie (1971, pp. 9ff.), this doctrine emerged in England during the eleventh century and was applied to the mentally ill during the fourteenth century. Nonetheless, the church, the guilds, and the lords of the manors generally cared for the mentally ill until the seventeenth to nineteenth centuries when there was a marked shift to predominately state guardianship.

In addition to those who may be dangerous to others, the community commits people who seem dangerous to themselves. The compassion involved in commitment of these individuals is much less obscured by outrage. Because society wishes to prevent them from doing something to themselves that may be irreversible and that they would not wish to do if they were in their right minds, they are protected (parens patriae). And if they do not wish this protection, once again the incompetence standard is invoked and their refusal of help is seen as a *product of mental illness*.

Some psychiatrists (e.g. Shah, 1975; Stone, 1976, Chapter 4) have rejected dangerousness as a suitable criterion for commitment, and many states do not employ it. Instead, some jurisdictions allow a person to be committed if he or she is "mentally ill and in need of care or treatment". In other words, severe mental illness is sufficient justification to abridge the right to be left alone. And in contrast with serious physical illness, the mentally ill person is not allowed to refuse the compassion of the State because he or she is felt not to be competent to make that decision. The State compassionately intervenes to prevent a foolish choice.

Regardless of which social aspect justification of commitment is employed, commitable individuals generally are distinguished from people in similar circumstances by the fact that they are not competent to consider the offer of help. (There are some recent exceptions to this principle, which are examined in Chapter Ten.) The social aspects have captured the attention of psychiatrists and the general public. However, as Stone (1981) suggests, it is the incompetence aspect which is the cutting edge that should differentiate commitable sick people from others.

STANDARDS. Prior to the midtwentieth century, people whom the family and the psychiatrist felt were mentally ill and needed treatment usually were not given the option of refusing hospitalization. During the 1960s and early 1970s a distinct change occurred. This was the era of political dissent. Civil liberties and a concern about government oppression, so prominent in the thinking of the framers of the Bill of Rights, once again came to the forefront of political thinking. The balance of interests was tilting toward indifference; champions of the right to be left alone were increasingly vociferous (Halleck, 1980, pp. 119ff.). In 1966, the same Judge Bazelon who had forged the *product of mental illness* concept for the criminal law stated that while society may have an obligation to care for the mentally ill, it should be done with the least deprivation of liberty possible — the least restrictive alternative (*Lake v Cameron*, 1966).

In the ensuing years, civil libertarians succeeded in increasing the tilt away from compassion and toward indifference by mounting a campaign to narrow the circle of conditions that would qualify a person for commitment. Using the criminal law as a guideline, they promoted the concept that the mentally ill person had to be dangerous in order to be committed; harmless mentally ill people should be left alone. As Halleck (1980, p. 120) has pointed out, this was part of a strategy to eliminate involuntary hospitalization altogether, because dangerousness in any particular case cannot be predicted with any acceptable level of accuracy (Dershowitz, 1969; Stone, 1976, Chapter 2). There are indications that by the 1980s the pendulum may be swinging back toward compassion, with a de-emphasis of rigorous dangerousness requirements (Psychiatric News, January 21, 1983).

These fluctuations in the standards referred only to the social aspect of the standards. The underlying implication that commitable people are those who are incompetent to make decisions about their hospitalization remained unstated. However, in 1976, Stone (pp. 66ff.) proposed a set of criteria that made the incompetence aspect explicit. (1) There must be a diagnosable, severe mental illness. (2) The patient is expected imminently to suffer major distress if not treated. (3) Appropriate treatment is available. (4) The "person [is] either too disturbed to communicate, or because of incapacity arising from the illness such as delusions or hallucinations, the person [is] unable to comprehend the possibility of treatment." (5) A reasonable person would not reject such treatment.

Based on Stone's proposal, the American Psychiatric Association issued guidelines for commitment standards in 1983 (APA, 1983) in which the social aspect included dangerousness for emergency commitment and dangerousness and the possibility of treatment for commitment up to thirty days. The incompetence aspect was stated explicitly in both the emergency and nonemergency situations.

Society's policymakers can accommodate changes in the balance of compassion and indifference by altering either the social or the incompetence aspect of the standards. The social aspect may be drawn narrowly by limiting the mental illnesses which qualify. Stone and the APA attempted to do this by referring to *severe* mental illness (which the APA defined as substantial impairment). As noted in Chapter Six, this is not effective. The social aspect can also be limited by such requirements as dangerousness, the possibility of treatment, the absence of alternatives to hospitalization, etc. On the other hand, the social aspect could be drawn broadly in burst of the parens patriae spirit to require only a mental illness for which the individual needs care.

The incompetence aspect could be broadened or narrowed by the types of mental illness that qualify and by the specific mental functions described. For example, Stone's proposals require the refusal of hospitalization to result from delusions or hallucinations—a cognitive standard. The APA guidelines allow more people to be declared incompetent by wording which could permit emotion and urge functions as well.

Both aspects of the standards require the decision maker to perform transductions. The social aspect requires a judgement of mental illness. Further, if there is a requirement of dangerousness, however defined, there is an implication that the dangerousness is a *product of mental illness*. Again, a transduction is needed.

Special mention should be made of the concept of "need for treatment" if it appears in the social aspect of the standards. Psychiatric expertise allows professionals to judge whether treatment is appropriate; sometimes they may even predict reasonably what might happen if no treatment is given. However, need is a value judgement that goes beyond psychiatric expertise; the psychiatrist says the individual needs hospitalization and the individual disagrees.

The mental illness transduction is repeated in the incompetence aspect. And the implication that the refusal of hospitalization results from the mental illness again necessitates a *product* transduction.

What is the role of psychiatrists in the setting up of these standards? Policymakers should be informed about various types of mental illnesses and their courses and treatment. The role of hospitalization as well as the conditions of the available hospitals should be discussed. Psychiatrists should avoid claiming special expertise in predicting dangerousness, not only because they do not have this expertise to any significant degree but also because they should not encourage society to hold them responsible for their patients' unforseeable actions. Of course, it is entirely within their expertise to tell the policymakers how the mental health system might be affected if, for example, the criteria include dangerousness or exclude the requirement that treatment be available), however, it should be noted that these predictions may not necessarily be accurate (Faulkner et al., 1982).

Psychiatrists should not pretend to have special expertise in deciding which mental illnesses and functions should appear in the standards or whether criteria such as dangerousness, need for care, or need for treatment should be included; how large or small the circle of those who would not be allowed to refuse hospitalization should be is not a psychiatric decision. Doctors are not neutral in the struggle between competing societal interests; there is a strong bias toward compassion that may influence professional judgements. The ultimate decisions about which conditions justify abridging the right to be left alone should be left to society's policymakers.

DECIDING THE INDIVIDUAL CASE. In emergency situations,

usually involving dangerousness, the psychiatrist must double as society's representative. When the police officer or family member brings the individual to the hospital, a decision must be made quickly. Since psychiatric expertise is needed to give input to the mental illness and *product* questions of the commitment standards, it is most expeditious to allow the doctor on the scene to make the necessary transductions and resolve the emergency. However, all sorts of extraneous factors operate in the emergency room. Often, the examining psychiatrist is one of the least trained and most overworked in the profession because hospital emergency work is not deemed to be one of the profession's most desirable pursuits (Langsley, 1980). The decision to commit or not in a marginal case may depend on bed availability or whether the psychiatrist can tolerate the anxiety of dismissing a patient about whom there may be some lingering doubt. Since psychiatrists generally tilt toward compassion and because there is no special expertise in making the critical transductions, a decision maker more representative of society at large should be brought into the process as soon as is practical.

This general procedure is followed in most jurisdictions, with a judge acting as society's representative when the emergency is not present or has passed. Since there are vastly more commitment decisions than criminal insanity pleas, requiring a full-blown jury hearing would unduly clutter the court system and would be impractical.

It seems that in any hearing before society's representative, the testimony of the psychiatrist should follow the recommendations made in Chapter Six regarding the insanity defense, because the basic issues are the same. A one-transduction system with psychiatric testimony limited to the question of sufficient mental illness and relating the behaviors in question to it is preferable. However, the psychiatrist should not testify about "allocation of *product*" issues.

One might propose that the psychiatrist could make transductions at the hearing and that the judge could then make the ultimate transduction. This would be a two-transduction plan as outlined in Chapter Four. The problem is that while two transductions might work in the insanity defense because the jury is often suspicious of the psychiatrist who testifies in favor of the defense, it will not work in commitment law because the average judge is all too ready to defer to the psychiatrist. Many judges tend to ignore the arguments of patients and their attorneys. The judges' attitudes are that "medical matters should be left up to doctors." Because of this, even in a one-transduction system, society's representatives, whether judges, ombudsmen, or whomever, should receive special training in order to recognize when the sychiatrist is exceeding his or her expertise by making a transction.

While the discussion up to this point has been concerned with the process of entering the hospital, it should be apparent that the patient's condition is not expected to remain static. There must be a process of periodic review by society's representative, and the patient should be released from involuntary hospitalization when he or she no longer fits the standards.

HOSPITALIZATION OF POLITICAL DISSENTERS

COMPETING SOCIETAL INTERESTS. Psychiatric hospitalization of political dissenters could be considered either in this chapter or in Chapter Six. At times, dissenters are judged in the criminal courts, while at other times, civil procedures are used. Because the political issues are so prominent, this book will attempt to gain some distance by examining the *product* issues involved in the hospitalization of dissenters in the USSR.

Two features of Soviet ideology must be understood in order to grasp the competing societal interests. First, there is a high value on social conformity. The supremacy of the State and Marxist-Leninist ideology is taught to children in the schools and impressed on adults from every billboard and a unified newsmedia. Part of this teaching is the need to be alert to anticommunist propaganda. Second, since the ideology teaches that the Soviet state is constructed on scientific principles (Galach'yan, 1968), the only possible reasons for significant dissent must be due to outside agitators (subversive propagandists) or mental illness (Bukovsky, 1977).

Seen from this ideological vantage point, the competing societal interests seem straightforward enough. If the dissent reaches criminal proportions (as defined by the Soviet criminal codes), the issue is one of outrage-compassion. The offender may be judged responsible (criminal) or nonresponsible (mentally ill). It is a *sick or criminal?* question. If the dissent does not reach criminal proportions (or does not attract the interest of the State's criminal justice system), civil commitment standards may be invoked. It becomes a compassion—indifference issue: *sick or unwise?* It is unclear how criminal and civil dissent problems are distinguished. Problems may be handled informally on a local level in a manner similar to that of the role of the police described in Chapter Six except for cases that may attract national or international attention.

If the ideological vantage point is shifted and this process is viewed while standing on the bedrock of American rather than Soviet values, the competing interests take on a different hue. As discussed earlier, the rights of the individual are so much more important in the United States, and there has been a long-standing wariness of government demands for conformity. In addition, as stated in the First Amendment, freedom of speech, expanded to freedom of expression, is a fundamental right. Americans jealously guard their right to criticize the government. The actions of the dissenters, which in the USSR are seen as criminal or unwise, are seen in the United States as praiseworthy. The competing interests center around the right to be left alone; they are compassion—indifference issues asking the question, *sick or praiseworthy?*

STANDARDS. Bloch and Reddaway (1977, Chapters 5 and 6) have outlined the standards used in the USSR in cases of political dissent. Their historical account of criminal commitment in the Soviet Union (pp. 97ff.) illustrates how the standards change with the temper of the times. The early postrevolutionary society tended to consider that "crime was basically a sociomedical problem, a result of the injustice and inequity of the tsarist regime." The tilt was toward compassion. During the 1930s, the social emphasis was more concerned with "saboteurs," "subversives," and "enemies of the State"; the tilt was toward outrage, and persons who committed "socially dangerous" offenses had little opportunity to be considered insane. Indeed, by 1945, psychiatric texts were stating that psychopathy is not a mental illness; therefore psychopaths were responsible for their actions (compare with the discussion of sociopathy in Chapter Two). As the atmosphere of extreme concern with counterrevolutionary activities relaxed following Stalin's death, the tilt toward outrage lessened and once again, dissenters could be deemed mentally ill.

The standards for criminal commitment of a person doing a "socially dangerous" act include (a) a mental illness, (b) because of this illness, an inability to realize the significance of this action, or (c) because of this illness, an inability to control his or her actions. Thus, the standards are very similar to the ALI standards described in Chapter Six. The civil commitment standards relevant to the dissenter issue are (a) mentally ill and (b) dangerous to those around him or her because of this illness. As in the American standards, neither the civil nor the criminal standards define a threshold mental illness.

As they stand in the law, there is little difference between the Soviet and the American standards. In terms of the social policies these standards reflect, however, there are three areas of substantial difference. The first difference is in the definition of danger, or "social danger." It is a difference in basic ideology important enough in itself but not a *product* issue.

The second difference is in what the professional and the social policymakers consider to be mental illnesses. Two diagnoses are of interest with respect to the hospitalization of dissenters: sluggish schizophrenia and paranoid development of the personality (Bukovsky and Gluzman, 1974; Bloch and Reddaway, 1977, Chapter 8). Sluggish schizophrenia is considered an indolent or slowly developing form of the illness in which there is a withdrawal of interest, development of pessimistic outlook, rigidity of outlook, suspiciousness and introspection. Rejection of traditions and standards may, but need not be, part of the picture. Bloch and Reddaway (pp. 244ff.) point out some similarities between this diagnosis and the American and British diagnoses of latent, borderline, and pseudoneurotic schizophrenia in use until recently.

People with paranoid development of the personality (paranoid psychopathy) show some grandiosity, a constriction of interests focussed on the area of their delusions, overevaluation of their ideas, and suspiciousness. The delusions may involve a conviction that they know the method for reform and improvement of society, or they may be of a different nature. These people may be prone to litigation. From the limited description that is available, there are some similarities to the category of paranoid personality disorder.

Whether these two diagnostic categories constitute mental illnesses and, if so, whether they should be considered threshold mental illnesses for criminal nonresponsibility or involuntary hospitalization are *product* issues. The position taken in this book is that they are not questions of fact but of policy; they should be left to society's policymakers. Psychiatrists may argue within their expertise whether sluggish schizophrenia has enough in common with other schizophrenic conditions to be usefully lumped with them; however, whether this cluster of characteristics should be called illness is beyond expertise.

The third difference is in the area of procedural safeguards of the individual's rights. This will be discussed in the following section.

DECIDING THE INDIVIDUAL CASE. According to Bloch and Reddaway (Chapter Five), in the criminal cases, the investigators (often the KGB) or the court sets up a commission of psychiatrists to report whether the individual fits the standards. The investigators or court may agree with the report, disagree with it, or ask for another report from a new commission. This is a two-transduction system with society's representatives having the final say. With respect to the *product* issues, then, it is similar to the system used in the United States, although the adversary system and the whole concept of due process (the legal system) is vastly different. In the civil commitment situation (Bloch and Reddaway, 1977, Chapter 6) one psychiatrist may admit a person to a hospital, and the commitment is reviewed by a panel of three psychiatrists. Essentially, this is a one-transduction system, which, in my view, relies on psychiatrists to make social judgements without judicial review.

This assumes there are impartial courts and conscientious psychiatrists; serious questions have been raised about both by Bloch and Reddaway and others. The conduct of the courts and investigators is beyond the scope of this book. Bukovsky and

Gluzman (1974) have described a variety of types of psychiatrists in the USSR. This book, however, will consider only the *Hangman* and the *Philistine*. The Hangman essentially is selling his or her opinions to the State and is aware that he or she is doing so. When Hangmen diagnose threshold mental illness, they are not making *product* decisions; they are choosing between outrage with one form of punishment (jail) and outrage with another form of punishment (incarceration in a Special Forensic Psychiatric Hospital), or in the case of civil commitment, between outrage and indifference. These are not *sick or* _____? questions because the compassion is only a sham. This type of situation will be discussed further in Chapter Ten. When Hangmen recommend that people with only mild schizophrenic symptoms need to be locked up in Special Forensic Psychiatric Hospitals instead of using less restrictive measures—in a country that boasts of an extensive network of outpatient facilities, there is no question of psychiatric expertise; it appears rather to be a matter of social expediency. It should not be surprising to find courts and investigators favoring commissions composed of Hangmen.

The Philistine is a rather unimaginative social conformist who, having been schooled in Soviet ideology and psychiatry, sincerely diagnoses dissenters as mentally ill. Philistines make *product* decisions wearing the dual hats of expert and society's representative. During his recent visit to the USSR, Reich (1983) gained the impression that the diagnostic scheme under which many Soviet dissenters are hospitalized has become standard throughout the country and that psychiatry as a discipline is particularly vulnerable to social conditioning.

Every country has its Hangmen, its Philistines, and all the other types of psychiatrists described by Bukovsky and Gluzman. Finding them in one country does not justify their existance in other countries. It is not difficult to judge the Hangmen; however, judging the Philistines is more difficult. The Philistine, making an honest though value-laden transduction, is doing procedurally what psychiatrists do everywhere.

I do not find fault with Soviet psychiatry because Philistines make value-laden transductions; all transductions everywhere are value laden. However, criticisms center around the societal values that prevent the profession from vigorous debate and self-scrutiny regarding the issue of political dissent. While there are disagreements with the Szaszes and Marcuses in the United States, the fact that they can speak out is healthy for the psychiatric profession and American society. My criticism of the Soviet system centers around the procedures by which the transductions are made—procedures that do not allow for vigorous debate and disagreement so that when the individual case is decided, both sides of the balance of competing interests are pressed. Not infrequently, some American psychiatrists grow impatient with the adversary system as it intrudes into psychiatric practice. Nonetheless, where transductions are involved, some potential for adversary process is the best guarantee not only against cultural Hangmen but also against the cultural Philistines who may misguidedly confuse social policy with psychiatric expertise.

REFUSING TREATMENT IN MENTAL HOSPITALS

COMPETING SOCIETAL INTERESTS. The fact that a person involuntarily has been placed in a hospital does not automatically deprive him or her of all individual rights. Not infrequently, such a patient decides not to accept the treatment offered in the hospital (*Rennie u Klein,* 1981; *Rogers u Okin,* 1980). A person's right to be left alone when others wish to force treatment has been justified on the grounds of a right to "bodily integrity" (Cantor, 1973) and a right not to have "unjustified intrusions on personal security" (*Ingraham u Wright,* 1977). Common law has long held that "every human being of adult years and sound mind has a right to determine what shall be done with his own body" (*Scholendorf u Society of New York Hospitals,* 1914). Treating someone without informed and voluntary consent has been considered battery.

The possible Constitutional bases for a right to refuse psychiatric treatment have been reviewed by Hansen and Plotkin (1977) and Stone (1981). Involuntary treatment has been considered to be an invasion of the right to privacy. In *Kaimowitz u Department of Mental Health* (1973) the court considered it an abridgement of freedom of expression (treatment that affects the mind may affect the freedom to generate ideas). Some treatments might be considered cruel and unusual punishment and thus violative of the Eighth Amendment.

In addition to the substantive legal considerations, undesirable side effects of treatment support society's interest in leaving the patient alone (Gaughn and LaRue, 1978). Medication side effects range from the annoying (e.g. dry mouth, lactation in women, weight gain) to various degrees of disability (e.g. temporary or permanent muscle dyscontrol, fatigue, sedation, confusion, sexual difficulties) to life endangering conditions (e.g. inability to fight off infections, heart problems, poor body temperature control). It is important to keep these side effects in mind because many patients refuse medications not because they fail to recognize they are ill but because they do not like the side effects.

Medication, with its risks, is not the only form of psychiatric treatment, of course. The array of therapeutic interventions ranges from psychotherapy to structured work tasks to relaxation or assertiveness training to aversive conditioning (training the patient to avoid inappropriate behaviors by making him or her feel extremely unpleasant whenever the behavior is performed) to physical restraint and seclusion to electroshock treatments to brain surgery. Each of these modalities has its own degree of risk, unpleasantness, and intrusiveness. The higher the degree of these factors, the greater the need for caution. However, the issue in risk intrusiveness is one of appropriateness or necessity of the high risk-intrusive treatment. It is not an issue that requires a decision about whether the patient's behavior is a *product of mental illness*. Therefore, although important, this area is beyond the scope of this book.

Counterbalancing the justifications for avoiding enforced treatment, there are arguments justifying the abridgement of the right to be left alone when the individual is in the mental hospital (Applebaum and Gutheil, 1980a and b, 1981). Once again, there are social and incompetence aspects to these justifications. The social criteria (which trigger interest in the process) can be classified in terms of parens patriae, police power, and economic justifications.

The basic parens patriae justification for enforced treatment is quite straightforward. Society has compassion for sick people and wants to help them. As in the case of mental hospitalization, the justification for treating mental patients differently from those with nonmental illnesses should rest on a finding of incompetence to make their own treatment decisions.

The police power justification in treatment refusal has to do not only with dangerousness but also with public health and welfare. Treatment is seen as a way of protecting staff and other patients from the harm that may be done by a highly agitated psychotic person. In addition to the possibility of danger, however, highly excited patients may create a disturbance that is inimical to the health and welfare of others on the ward (Applebaum and Gutheil, 1981). Loud singing at night, constant disruption of others' conversations, inability to conform to the basic rules necessary for close group living not only may irritate other patients and impede their recovery, but also may command an inordinate amount of time and attention from staff at the expense of the needs of others. The ability of the hospital to provide health care may deteriorate significantly. Voluntary patients, of course, could be discharged; the hospital is stuck with committed patients.

There is a third area of justification for overriding the patient's desire to refuse treatment—economics. Although rarely made explicit, it lurks behind many, many decisions that are made within hospital walls. The need of the hospitalized patient for medication, especially on an emergency basis, is often rooted in the total situation on the ward. There are some data which suggest that disputes about treatment may diminish if the hospital has adequately trained staff and a milieu philosophy which is conducive to cooperation (Bursten and Geach, 1976). Many of the mental hospitals scandalously are underfunded and have such thin and poorly trained staff that they cannot even meet accreditation standards. In such a situation, medication often is given not for compassionate reasons but to keep peace and order while placing minimal demands on staff. It is cheaper to buy medicine than to hire professionals. In a sense, the right to refuse medication is overbalanced by the need to save money (Bursten et al., 1980). This issue will be further considered in Chapter Ten.

STANDARDS. For many years, the right of the hospital's doctors to treat involuntary patients went virtually undisputed. In several states, commitment automatically transferred decisionmaking to the next of kin or to the superintendent. The same social and political forces that promoted the rights of individuals to refuse mental hospitalization in the 1960s and 1970s promoted a reconsideration of the hospitalized patient's right to refuse treatment.

Indeed, the social situations (parens patriae and police power) that trigger enforced treatment are roughly the same as those that trigger commitment. Thus, it would be reasonable to construct the social aspect of the standard for enforced treatment as broadly or narrowly as the social aspect of the commitment standard. (The economic justification is not a *product* issue and does not lend itself to a standard. Thus, while it should be of the greatest concern as a public scandal, it is not of primary concern in this chapter.)

Where the commitment standard does not include incompetence, this aspect should be added to the standard for involuntary treatment. In most of the standards currently in use, incompetence is the cornerstone of the decision to override the refusal of treatment. In general, the standards of incompetence used in mental hospitals are similar to those proposed in the APA (1983) guidelines: A person who "lacks capacity to make an informed decision concerning treatment [is one who], by reason of his mental disorder or condition, is unable despite conscientious effort at explanation to understand basically the nature and effect of . . . treatment, or is unable to engage in a rational decision-making process regarding such . . . treatment as evidenced by inability to weigh the possible risks and benefits." While this appears to be a cognitive standard, it easily could be interpreted more broadly to include emotive or urge functions that may be felt to impair the ability to weigh the possible risks and benefits.

If the commitment standards and the involuntary treatment standards both have the same social and incompetence aspects, it might make sense not to have two sets of standards at all. Commitment can be considered as one (very restrictive) form of treatment. If the individual's behavior meets the social criterion and he or she lacks competence to form treatment decisions at the time of commitment, these judgements could cover other types of treatments as well. All committed patients could be treated involuntarily. Utah (UCA 6407-36 [10]) has a procedure similar to this.

This suggestion should not be interpreted as giving the psychiatrist carte blanche to use any treatment measures he or she wishes. As noted, there are still more or less risky and intrusive forms of treatment, and the greater the risk intrusiveness, the more stringent should be the monitoring. This, however, is not a *product* issue.

If the patient is in the hospital and no longer meets the commitment standards, he or she should be uncommitted and converted to voluntary status. The next section shall consider what should be done when a voluntary patient refuses treatment.

DECIDING THE INDIVIDUAL CASE. Two social situations have a significant impact on the decision process in the individual case: emergency versus nonemergency and voluntary patient versus involuntary. The role of the psychiatrist as decisionmaker will vary along these parameters.

There are essentially two types of emergencies on the psychiatric ward. In one type, the patient is imminently likely to suffer a serious deterioration. This is a psychiatric judgement, and if this type of emergency is written into the standard, it is reasonable that the psychiatrist decide if the patient fits. The second type of emergency is that of danger to others and it requires that the decisionmaker establish that such danger is a *product of mental illness.* In such as emergency situation, it is reasonable that the psychiatrist act also as society's representative and allocate the *product* between the sick and healthy aspects of the person's mental functioning. However, it is important to bear in mind what situations could give rise to nonsick outbursts and threats. At times, hospitals that are thinly staffed with untrained personnel can be unduly oppressive toward patients; obedience, peace, and quiet may be demanded. A patient who is being treated unfairly by staff or by other patients in the absence of adequate staff supervision may rebel not because of mental illness but because of justified anger. In terms of the sociology of the ward, doctors tend to try to accommodate the wishes of the nursing staff with whom they must work. Therefore, there is the possibility that the psychiatrist might be prone to see too many danger situations as *products of mental illness.* For that reason, if a patient is treated against his or her wishes because of imminent danger, there should be some automatic mechanism of review by a more neutral observer. It would be far too expensive to do this on a case by case basis; however, periodic reviews of the practices of units with high frequencies of dangerous emergencies would be feasible and desirable.

The situation vis-à-vis voluntary versus involuntary patients has already been discussed. Only incompetent patients should be committed, and the social aspects of the involuntary treatment standard should be the same as those of the commitment standard. Thus, there would be no *product* decision to be made at the time treatment is recommended. Voluntary patients should never be treated against their wishes; they should be discharged if it is felt that without the offered treatment, no progress can be made. However, there is often more than one way to approach treatment; discharge should not be used as a threat to force consent to intrusive treatments. Again, some method of review would be desirable.

What about the voluntary patient whose sudden deterioration constitutes an emergency? Obviously, there is no time to have society's representative listen to the input of the psychiatrist and decide if the patient is incompetent. The psychiatrist must make the decision. However, it seems that this situation should trigger an emergency commitment procedure. Once again, if the patient is competent to refuse one form of treatment, he or she should be competent to refuse all. If the psychiatrist is treating the patient against his or her wishes and simultaneously feels that the patient cannot be discharged as an alternative, the requirements of commitment are met. This procedure would have the safeguard of invoking the subsequent review and protections outlined in the section on commitment.

REFUSING TREATMENT FOR NONMENTAL ILLNESSES

COMPETING SOCIETAL INTERESTS. The societal interests in protecting the right to refuse general medical treatment are essentially the same as those described in the section on refusal of psychiatric treatment: The integrity of one's privacy and bodily security and the common law principle that unauthorized touching of another person constitutes battery. In addition, protection of freedom of religious belief has at times nurtured this right (*In re Osborne*, 1972).

Dangerousness to others and disruptiveness which formed part of the justification for abridging the right to refuse psychiatric treatment is not a factor in other medical settings. For example, respiratory illnesses such as lung cancer do not result in these types of behaviors unless the disease has spread to the brain. At this point, the disruptive behavior is an issue of mental illness (often delirium). Even if the patient remains on the medical or surgical ward, if treatment for the mental illness is refused, he or she should be treated according to the guidelines in the preceding section.

Most often, however, dangerous or disruptive behavior is not the trigger for the dispute. Rather, the interest in treating the patient is a compassionate and straightforward parens patriae interest; society wishes to preserve life and health. In addition, there is a long social and religious tradition of preventing people from taking their own lives.

STANDARDS. Special cases, such as treatment of life-threatening emergencies, refusal of treatment on religious grounds, or the preparation of a living will (outlining the conditions under which a person wishes to be allowed to die if he or she should contract a terminal illness) pose special problems for society's policy makers, but since they do not involve psychiatric decisionmaking, they will not be considered here.

The sole product situation in the refusal of general medical treatment is incompetence. The standard has been defined in the previous section. What commands special attention in these cases is the fact that there often has been no previous question of mental illness. The inability to weigh the risks and benefits of the treatment may not be based on delusions but on beliefs or fears. It is up to the decision maker to say whether such beliefs or fears are the *product of mental illness* rather than cultural myths.

DECIDING THE INDIVIDUAL CASE. Not infrequently, colleagues in the other medical specialties expect that psychiatrists will determine that their patient is incompetent and give them permission to proceed with treatment. Psychiatrists cannot do this, nor should they be able to do so. Incompetence, as a *product* decision, is beyond psychiatric expertise. Professionals can evaluate the patient, make a diagnosis, point out what mental functions the patient displays that are consistent with that diagnosis, and (perhaps) make their own transduction. However, the ultimate allocations and transductions must be made by society's representative, usually a judge.

Two problems are likely to arise when the psychiatrist makes the transduction on the general medical patient. The first is the problem of bias. As mentioned earlier, doctors have a strong bias toward compassion and, especially in cases of serious illness, might tend to feel that most objections to treatment are irrational. Further, just as physicians often will give in to the wishes of the nursing staff with which they work, a specialist has a tendency to accommodate the wishes and needs of the doctor who referred the patient for consultation. These factors often operate in a subtle way and the psychiatrist may not even be aware of them.

The second problem occurs in the case of patients with chronic deteriorating illnesses who wish to end their suffering by dying. Indeed, some of them truly may be depressed in reaction to their condition. Does that make the decision a *product of mental illness* and render the patient incompetent? The answer to this question lies beyond the expertise of the psychiatrist and should be referred to a representative of society.

THE DESIRE OF THE ELDERLY
TO MANAGE THEIR OWN AFFAIRS

COMPETING SOCIETAL INTERESTS. Guardianship of the mentally ill has existed since ancient Rome (Brakel and Rock, 1971, Chapter 1). The aged person for whom guardianship is assigned may lose decision-making powers over property disposal, finances, purchases, driving, voting, medical treatment, and even place of residence and freedom of movement (Schmidt et al., 1981, p. 10). These losses of the right to be left alone touch on many of the fundamental societal interests described earlier in this chapter. In addition to the constitutionally derived rights that are abridged, the individual may suffer a loss of adult status, loss of opportunities, and denial of pleasures. He or she may have to submit to the whim and personality of the guardian. This may be an overworked public guardian whose tastes and standards can be quite different from those of the person in question. There is also the possibility that the guardian who is a family member may have a desire to exploit the ward while doing as little as possible for him or her. All of these factors tilt towards indifference—allowing the aged to make their own decisions.

However, society also has compassion for some of the aged who may be incompetent to make their own decisions (Schmidt et al., 1981, pp. 146ff.). They also may be subject to exploitation and even abuse and neglect at the hands of unscrupulous acquaintances or relatives. While some of the aged merely need good advice, society feels that some need protection.

STANDARDS. Decisions of the aged have been selected as an example of the many situations where an individual is deprived of the right to make his or her own decisions. This will give the reader an opportunity to consider some general problems in this area. Remarks will be confined to mental incompetence. The standards of incompetence used in Tennessee are typical of those used generally.

Tennessee has a limited guardianship law (TCA 34-12-101–118) that can deprive the individual of any or all of the areas previously denoted. The deprivations are written in the disjunctive. This illustrates a basic rule about incompetence: Incompetence to make decisions in one area does not necessarily mean incompetence in all areas. Each area of decision making must be separately tested.

What are the standards by which incompetence in these areas are tested? The report to the court must include the following: the person's medical history, "a description of the nature and type of the respondent's disability," a recommendation about guardianship with the reasons for such recommendation, and anything else of importance. These instructions set no standards at all.

In practice, each area is scrutinized for three things: mental illness, a cognitive test of understanding in the specific area as discussed at the beginning of this chapter, and evidence of recent behavior based on decisions felt to be inappropriate. The existence of mental illness requires a transduction; this becomes a problem especially in close calls. If the person fails to understand the nature and consequences of the decision, society is still faced with the task of attributing the failure to the mental illness (an allocation problem). Likewise, even if psychiatrists can agree to call the recent behavior inappropriate, it requires a transduction to attribute it to the mental illness.

There is another subtle aspect to the standards that creeps in when considering recent behavior. Even if the individual currently shows a good cognitive grasp of the issues in any particular area, if he or she has recently made an inappropriate decision in that area because of an overwhelming emotional state or because of impulsivity, the person is likely to be declared incompetent. Despite the apparent cognitive limits on the tests, emotional and urge functions are also considered.

DECIDING THE INDIVIDUAL CASE. Who should make these decisions? It does not take a psychiatrist to test whether the person's recent behavior was inappropriate; indeed the psychiatrist relies on reports of family members, etc. for this information. Nor is a psychiatrist necessary to test whether the person can understand the issues in any particular area. The psychiatrist is needed only to state whether the behavior and/or the lack of understanding is a *product of mental illness.* And that is precisely what lies beyond psychiatric expertise, because it requires transductive activity. These are squarely the dilemmas discussed in Chapters Two and Three. And, as mentioned in those chapters, the dilemmas may not matter when the illness is blatant and the decision is bizarre; however, in these cases, one does not need a psychiatrist at all, except to lend credence to what everyone can plainly see. It is in the disputed cases, the close calls, that the *product* dilemmas may come painfully to the forefront.

From the standpoint of the *product* issues, the situation is precisely the same as in criminal responsibility, and it should not be surprising that the decision making is also the same. Currently, a two-transduction system is used; the psychiatrist transduces in formulating a recommendation of incompetence and the judge transduces in agreeing or disagreeing. And, as in the case of criminal responsibility, the system might be improved and the psychiatrist kept more nearly within the bounds of his or her expertise if a one-transduction system similar to that outlined in Chapter Four were used.

For many years, psychiatrists such as Menninger, (1966, pp. 139ff.), Halleck (1967), and Zilboorg (1968, pp. 112ff.), have been warning psychiatrists not to make moral and social pronouncements dressed in medical clothes when testifying whether a defendant in criminal court had the capacity to choose his or her actions. It is striking that the psychiatric community has not been concerned equally about the ability to state whether a person is incompetent since the *product* dilemmas are the same. Part of the reason for this difference, of course, is that psychiatry has been embarrassed by conflicting expert testimony in the criminal courtroom; public exposure of the conceptual difficulty in *product* decisions has not been so prominent in incompetence cases. However there probably is an additional reason for this difference. In the criminal setting, the tension is between compassion and outrage and psychiatrists are not supposed to be the arbiters of outrage. In incompetence proceedings, the tension is between compassion and indifference; it is as if the question were, "Is the individual sick or not?" This would seem more like a question to ask the doctor. Society tends to forget that the *not* is not an absence of something but a bona fide attitude that society will take toward the individual.

THE DECISION TO HAVE RHINOPLASTY

Before leaving the area of the right to be left alone when making one's own decisions, one area of potential confusion will be discussed. At times, when the individual decides to do something that another person disallows because it would be unwise, it is not a *product* situation at all. For example, a person may wish to have an operation to change the shape of his or her nose (rhinoplasty), and the plastic surgeon may request a psychiatric consultation. The psychiatrist may advise against the operation because the patient exhibits mental characteristics that make him or her a high risk for unfortunate psychiatric sequellae of the surgery (Goin and Goin, 1981). This is not a question of incompetence to make a decision; the psychiatrist is not saying that the patient's decision is a *product of mental illness*. The psychiatrist is relying on data and experience arrived at in the deterministic mode in order to make a prediction; these characteristics may have a likelihood of such an outcome after surgery. This is properly within the realm of psychiatric expertise.

Interestingly enough, the plastic surgeon is not really interested in whether the patient is mentally ill. If the psychiatrist responds only with a diagnosis, the plastic surgeon has not been given the help needed. What the surgeon wants is some estimate of psychiatric risk; whether the risk factors are called *illness* is irrelevant.

The plastic surgeon may decline to do the operation, not because the patient was incompetent, but because the operation was too risky. This predictive type of situation must be distinguished from those where the right to make one's own decisions is abridged because of incompetence. Only the incompetence situation involves a *product* decision.

CHAPTER EIGHT

COMPASSION—INDIFFERENCE

The Desire To Be Designated Sick

In the previous chapter, immunities and claims were differentiated. Immunity is the right to be left alone, to be free from others' intervention in one's affairs. A claim is the expectation of something from others; if valid, it imposes a duty on the other person or agency to do something for the individual (Hohfeld, 1919). In the immunity situation, it is usually the other person or agency that initiates the action; in the claim situation, the action generally is initiated by the individual in question. Chapter Seven dealt with immunity—the right to be treated with indifference. The present chapter deals with claims—the desire to be treated with compassion. In the conflict situations to be discussed below, certain agencies wish to treat the individual with indifference while the individual, citing mental illness, wishes to be treated in some special way by these agencies.

There are two types of situations in which the person wishes to be designated sick: claims of exemption and claims of entitlement. In claims of exemption, the individual takes the position that mental illness prevents him or her from doing what others are expected to do. Examples are the wish to retract a confession of a crime (Bursten, 1979b), to nullify a signed contract, to invalidate a marriage, or to challenge a will on the grounds that the testator was of unsound mind. In the school situation, the person may wish to delay an exam or to take a leave of absence. In the workplace, the individual may attempt to escape reprimand for poor performance or to take sick leave because of mental illness. One could easily think of other exemption situations. The nullification of contracts and the request for a leave of absence from school will be considered as illustrations of two subtypes of claims of exemption.

Claims of entitlement state that a person or agency has the affirmative duty to provide something for the individual because of his or her mental illness. Examples are disability claims, workers' compensation, mental sequellae of personal injuries (e.g. accidents, major disasters, or sexual harrassment), special school classes for the emotionally disturbed, the request for treatment, etc. Social security disability, personal injury claims, and the request for treatment also will be considered as examples of claims of entitlement.

EXEMPTIONS

Nullifying a Contract

COMPETING SOCIETAL INTERESTS. American society places great emphasis on both the freedom to contract and the importance that contracts be kept. Judge Jessel (*Printing and Numerical Registration Co. u Sampson*, 1875) said, "[I]f there is one thing which, more than any other, public policy requires, it is that men of full age and competent understanding shall have the utmost liberty of contracting . . . " This right to contract fosters personal autonomy and fulfills an important economic function (Green, 1940). However, these interests are realized only if the contract is sustained over time. If an individual breaks the contract or causes it to be invalidated, he or she is abridging the right of the other party. The other party may suffer material loss by way of missed opportunities and emotional consequences such as disappointment and potential further problems in arranging a new contract with another party. If too many contracts were invalidated, public trust in the value of contracts would be weakened and the economic system would be undercut. These factors, based on the concept that the parties freely chose to make the agreement, tilt the balance toward indifference; even if one party wishes to get out of the contract, society has a tendency not to want to interfere with it.

On the other hand, Green (1940) cites some interests society may have in allowing a contract to be invalidated. The legal concept of a contract requires a "meeting of the minds" — minds that are intact and able to give free and informed consent. Legal transactions are governed by the concept that both parties should be equal, and the law guards that equality by protecting someone who may be a "mental underdog." This, of course, is a parens patriae view; compassion dictates that society should not allow a mentally disadvantaged person to suffer. Further, there is a strong bias in society to protect the family unit. Compassion for the individual spreads to his or her family who might suffer if the contract might waste its economic resources.

STANDARDS. Nullifying a contract (and other nullifications) hinges on an assessment of incompetence and thus the issues are similar to those discussed in the preceding chapter. And, as in many incompetence situations, the standards are not particularly clear. Although the general standard had been a cognitive one (Did the party appreciate the nature and possible consequences of the contract?), in the wake of the *Durham* decision in the criminal area, broader standards started to creep into the civil law as well (Comment, 1964). *Faber u Sweet Style Mfg. Co.*, (1963) set a course for judging incompetence on the basis of urge functions, even when the cognitive test might have been passed. Isadore Faber, who suffered from bipolar affective illness, had entered a manic phase. Although usually "frugal and cautious, he became more expansive . . . , began to drive at high speeds, to take his wife out to dinner(!), to be sexually more active, and to discuss his prowess with others. In a short period of time, he purchased three expensive cars . . . " He began imprudently buying up real estate to fulfill his grandiose plans. All parties agreed that when he contracted to buy the Sweet Style Manufacturing Co., Mr. Faber understood what he was doing. He even bargained down the price. However, the contract was subsequently nullified on the grounds that Mr. Faber, because of his mental illness, could not control his impulsiveness.

The *Restatement (Second) of Contracts* (1973) specifically suggested that a person may be incompetent to make a contract if "[he] lack[s] capacity to control his acts in the way that the normal individual can and does control them. . . . " Kowalski (1970) suggested that the new (urge) criteria does not limit contractual incompetence to psychotic people but might also include "severely neurotic people." Thus, the widest possible band of people might be found to have been incompetent when they signed contracts. What are the limits of incompetence sufficient to nullify contracts? They may be substantially left up to the decisionmakers.

DECIDING THE INDIVIDUAL CASE. The essential difference between decision making in nullification situations and in current activities, such as the desire of the elderly to make their own decisions, is that in nullifications, the mental state of the actor must be ascertained in retrospect. This poses certain problems and may limit the accuracy of data, but it does not pose a *product* dilemma.

As in the case of the desire of the elderly to make their own decisions, currently in operation is a two-transduction system in the nullification of decisions. The psychiatrist makes the transductions necessary to designate the existence of mental illness and the allocation of the product and so does society's decisionmaker, the judge, who has the final say. A one-transduction system as outlined in Chapter Four would better allow psychiatrists to stay within their own area of special expertise. It could, for example, establish whether people with diagnoses that fall in the severely neurotic range would qualify for nullification.

The Request for a Leave of Absence from College

COMPETING SOCIETAL INTERESTS. The situation considered here usually occurs when a student's grades in college have been going downhill. At times, this may be precipitous, as in the case of a psychotic decompensation; at other times it may extend over the better part of a semester. Often, the request for a leave of absence comes shortly before the final exam when the student anticipates a failing grade for the course. The behavior is not the decision to take a leave of absence; if that were the case, this would be an example of the incompetence situations reviewed in the preceding chapter. The behavior in question is that of not proceeding in college in the expected manner. The issue is whether this lack of continuing is because the person, by virtue of mental illness, *cannot* continue to do the work or whether he or she *chooses* not to do the work for any number of reasons, such as too many outside distractions or a lack of perseverance. It is a *sick or lazy?* or *sick or manipulative?* type of situation. In Chapter Five, the problem of detecting manipulativeness (malingering) was considered and shall not be further discussed at this point. The college administration may turn to the psychiatrist for help with the *sick or lazy?* question.

The college has certain interests in not granting leaves of absence. One of the tasks of college education is to help the adolescent mature into an autonomous and independent adult. If it grants exemptions for frivolous reasons, it undercuts the effort to turn out responsible adults. In this sense, the school's interest in the development of its students may require an attitude of indifference in terms of not wishing to intervene in the usual course of things.

Besides its interest in the students, the college must guard its own interests in maintaining the institution. Colleges are empowered by tradition and by law to use procedures that enable them to continue to function effectively (Bakken, 1970). If too many people take leaves of absence, the school may have difficulty planning classes and schedules. A relatively small school or one with a single orderly curriculum could find next year's classes clogged with students returning from this year's leaves. Colleges have limited resources. A student who comes back next year to repeat courses taken before he or she dropped out may be seen as using up resources that could be spent on other students. Colleges also have what might be called a productivity task. They are charged with turning out graduates who have completed the requirements and gained an education. Student leaves of absence interfere with this productivity. While it is true that employee leaves of absence in college or industry create a greater interference and added cost, student leaves do result in a delay of the product. For all these reasons, colleges have an interest in keeping the number of leaves of absence down to a minimum.

On the other hand, colleges do have compassion for their sick students. Along with society's general swing toward compassion in the 1950s (described in Chapter Six), colleges took on expanded obligations to help with emotional problems. There was a virtual explosion of student counselling and mental health services (Pearlman, 1968). Approximately 0.2 percent to 0.3 percent of students become actively psychotic during their college years (Farnsworth, 1966, p. 51); nearly 10 percent of all college students have emotional difficulties serious enough to warrant professional intervention (Pearlman, 1968; Whitley, 1979). The college has already invested some of its resources in these students and experience teaches that many of them can complete the course of education and become valuable assets to society at large (Group for the Advancement of Psychiatry [GAP], 1957). Thus, there is a general trend for colleges to do their best to provide conditions whereby matriculated students may complete their courses even if they take a leave of absence to accomplish it. Actually, many colleges tend to extend to their students the most liberal leave-taking opportunities.

There are occasionally other competing interests within the sociopolitical structure of the college. At times, the competition between compassion and indifference may reflect a turf battle between the dean (or committee) in charge of academic progress and the dean (or committee) responsible for student affairs. Academic progress people tend to identify more with the regulatory needs of the school while student affairs people tend to identify with the individual student. The request for a leave of absence may be the stage on which a power struggle is being enacted.

These, then, are some of the interests that make up the competition between compassion and indifference when the student expresses the desire to be designated sick in order to obtain a leave of absence from college. This is a *product* situation because the leave will be granted only if the noncontinuance is due to mental illness. It is an exemption situation inasmuch as the student wishes to be exempted from doing what others are expected to do. However, it should be differentiated from three other types of situations that seem closely related: admission to college, exemption from military service, and leave of absence versus disciplinary expulsion.

The admission of students who may be or may have been mentally ill is not a *product* issue at all. The issue is essentially that described in the previous chapter with regard to the desire to have a rhinoplasty. The student wants admission; his or her mental condition may constitute a risk factor for successful completion of the course. This is a predictive rather than a *product* situation; as such, it falls within the realm of psychiatric expertise.

An individual may wish to be exempted from a general military draft on the grounds of mental illness. Although an exemption situation, this is not a *product* issue; it is essentially the same as the rhinoplasty situation. The question is not whether the person is mentally ill but whether he or she exhibits risk factors which suggest that the performance in the military service will be substandard. As in the case of college admissions, this is a predictive situation that is a reasonable psychiatric endeavor. Admissions and military exemption are not essentially tugs between compassion and indifference. The tilt of the emotional tension is not (or should not be) the issue. Rather, the issue in these types of cases are matters of fact, at least to whatever degree research has yielded the pertinent facts: Have such people been shown in the past to do well or not to do well? However, being granted a leave of absence because of mental illness is a policy decision that rests on the balance between compassionate and indifferent interests.

The third type of situation that must be differentiated is the case where someone who has made a serious infraction of the disciplinary rules wishes a leave of absence on the grounds that his or her actions were due to mental illness. School officials, on the other hand, wish to expel the student. This is a compassion—outrage situation, similar to the insanity defense, rather than a compassion—indifference situation. It is a true *product* issue, the ultimate resolution of which should be left up to the representatives of the college.

STANDARDS. There are no standards to guide the decision maker in judging whether the desire to take a leave of absence is based on mental illness. Indeed, as might be expected, except in the case of blatant psychosis, there is dispute among professionals over whether many of the emotional upsets of college students should be designated as mental illness altogether. Nixon (1964) has argued that most of the disturbances do not fit into diagnostic categories, while Selzer (1960) has maintained that student mental health centers grossly underdiagnose those who come for help. The individual decision maker is left on his or her own, and this allows for the widest possible criteria to be employed by a decision maker who tends to be compassionate.

DECIDING THE INDIVIDUAL CASE. The individual student often has difficulty in studying because of an inability to concentrate. Three conditions will be considered: psychosis, depression, and other conditions. If the psychosis is blatant, there is often no issue to be decided. When the psychiatrist is consulted, it is only to legitimate a decision based on compassion that has already been made. If the psychosis is not obvious, the psychiatrist may detect it and discuss how a person preoccupied with delusions or bothered by hallucinations finds it difficult to concentrate. If the psychiatrist has a credible record (i.e. he or she does not have the reputation of stretching the truth as a means of oversympathizing with students), the decision probably will be in favor of the leave. The psychiatrist's role in this situation is one of diagnosis; there is no need to suggest a leave of absence. This means there is no need for the psychiatrist to make a transduction.

If the student has a significant clinical depression, the response should be similar to that in the case of psychosis—diagnosis and relevance to the problem in studying. There is one further consideration. The psychiatrist must attempt to determine if the depression was precipitated by the imminent scholastic failure or whether it occurred independently. If the student is depressed because he or she is failing, even though there is now a bona fide medical reason for the student's being unable to carry on with the work, the administration may decide to act with less compassion.

The other conditions are more difficult; they are the close calls. Here, the psychiatrist is not called on to legitimate a decision all agree upon. Instead, there may be disagreement based both on the competing interests and on the competition between academic progress people and student affairs people. The psychiatrist is invited to be an ally. This situation is not too different from the subtle forces found in other situations already described in this book. The difference is in the relative informality of the process. The psychiatrist can talk informally to both administrative groups about the limits of professional expertise. This informal discussion enables the psychiatrist to stick with a one-transduction procedure. The student can be described in terms of diagnosis and relevant specific mental functions. The administrators can be reminded that decisions about a leave of absence are up to them. The psychiatrist may add that if a leave is granted, the student should be reevaluated prior to resuming his or her studies. There is a logic to this: The psychiatrist does not have the expertise to state whether the close call should be designated as a *product of mental illness* justifying a leave of absence. However, when the student wishes to return, the psychiatrist may evaluate whether the conditions he or she had observed during the first evaluation have cleared up. If not, the administration may wish to take the position that conditions which justify absence cannot also justify resumption of studies. In all of this procedure, the psychiatrist is able to remain well within his or her area of expertise.

ENTITLEMENTS

Social Security Disability

COMPETING SOCIETAL INTERESTS. In the context of social security disability, the behavior in question is nonemployment. Essentially, when this nonemployment is determined to be a product of illness, the claimant is considered to be disabled and is entitled to benefits. Thus, this topic straddles both exemption (the person is excused from work) and entitlement (the person receives money from the federal government).

While there is some coherent theory of forces and ideals behind the insanity defense (see Chapter Six), society's posture toward social security has been marked by a hodgepodge of aims (Liebman, 1976). Policies have evolved as much in response to various pressure groups and discrete court decisions as to overriding social policy considerations. As Liebman indicates, society lacks a good theory to explain "why Smith is paid and Green is not."

Social security seems to have been conceived as a cross between a form of insurance against the time when one would be too old to work and a minimum income guarantee for those who are covered. As such, it expresses compassionate attitudes toward those who work. During the years since its inception in 1935, the concept evolved to offer benefits not only to those who could no longer work because of old age but also to those who could no longer work because of medical illness. However, as Liebman pointed out, for the person who has not reached the requisite old age, the compassion extends only to medical disability. Only the person who suffers "an involuntary decline in working capacity" is to be supported. Those who do not work because of laziness, unreliability, or surliness are not covered. Likewise, those who do not work because of external factors, such as a shrinking job market or technological unemployment, are not eligible for disability benefits (20 CTR 404.1566 [c]). Only the sick are singled out for that extra measure of compassion because they cannot help themselves.

This exception was carved out of a more general policy of indifference toward the unemployed. While there are a welter of welfare and unemployment insurance programs, the latter are temporary and the former carry a stigma that social security disability payments lack. Americans feel entitled to social security payments because they worked for them (the insurance aspect). Society places a high value on work; as Liebman indicated, "Those who can work must work." This provides the framework for the counterbalancing themes of indifference. There is the glorification of work, the social desire to foster independence and self-reliance, and the preference for self-paid insurance over government dole.

In addition to the social desire to promote the work and independence ethic, fiscal considerations tend to weigh the balance toward indifference. In 1981, nine out of ten men and five out of ten women between the ages of twenty-one and sixty-four were covered by social security (McCormick, 1983, p. 13). As seen in recent years, social security is a system under severe financial strain. Any policy towards disability that takes increasing numbers of people out of the work force where they pay into the system and puts them into the position of taking money out of the system increases the fiscal distress.

However, in contrast to many other *product* situations, social security is bolstered by an enormous political momentum that makes it less responsive to swings in the social mood. Because the benefits are felt to be earned, it is very difficult to curtail them when the mood of the country shifts. While the circle of people judged mentally ill in the insanity defense and commitment situations may expand and contract with the temper of the times, the social security disability circle may expand more easily than it contracts.

STANDARDS. As indicated in Chapter Four, the number of people who will be judged compassionately varies with shifts in the balance of competing societal interests. The guidelines for judging, whereby this adjustment is accomplished, consist of some considerations in addition to the *product of mental illness* standards. In the case of social security disability, such factors as defining the minimal length of time the person must have been disabled, controlling the payment schedules, altering the frequency of the periodic reviews of disability, etc. all serve to allow greater or fewer numbers of people to qualify for benefits. This book shall focus on the *product* standards, however.

Social security standards afford an excellent opportunity to examine many of the *product* issues because they represent a conglomerate of laws and court decisions that have had to be translated into regulations (20 CFR 404). Because it is an entitlement program sponsored by the federal government and because it must be administered on a day-to-day basis by many agencies all over the country, all the definitions, all the rules, and all the standards of evaluation are written down.

The first element of the standards, of course, is mental illness. The regulations (20 CFR 404 P. App. 1) list virtually the entire gamut of mental illness, albeit in DSM II rather than DSM III nomenclature. Chronic brain disorders, psychoses, neuroses, psychophysiological disorders, personality disorders and addictions all qualify. Even "psychological disability" (*Dressel u Califano,* 1977) and psychogenic pain and discomfort without sufficient objective findings which would make the "average person" have that much pain (*Thorne u Weinberger,* 1976) are included in the category of mental illnesses. About the only clusters of mental characteristics that are disqualified are sexual types and disorders, malingering, and disorders of adjustment to situational stresses; and all of these except malingering could be given appropriate accepted diagnoses. In other words, the basic diagnostic list is wide open.

The regulations require that the mental illness in question be a severe one. The concepts of severe and substantial mental illness have been encountered previously in Chapters Six and Seven, but the basic circularity of these concepts so blatantly expressed can be found nowhere as they are in the Social Security standards. The behavior in question is nonemployment. This behavior must be the result of a severe impairment. And what is a severe impairment? "If you do not have any impairment(s) which significantly limits your ... mental ability to do basic work activities, we will find that you do not have a severe impairment ... " (20 CFR 404.1520 [c]). Conversely, a nonsevere impairment is one that "does not significantly limit ... basic work activities," such as carrying out simple instructions, using judgement, "responding appropriately" to others on the job, and coping with changes at work (20 CFR 404.1521). In other words, unemployment is a *product of mental illness* when the mental illness is of the nature that makes it impossible to be employed.

Any *product* standard that requires a mental illness which is severe, substantial, serious, or any other adjective implying high degree is circular by its very nature. In this regard, the concept of "sufficient mental illness" (Chapter Four) has a different context, because sufficiency or threshold is defined not in quantitative terms but by diagnostic category.

However, elsewhere the regulations offer other qualifying criteria as well (20 CFR 404 P. App. 1). While they are behavioral descriptions, they can be considered as specific mental characteristics in the terms used in this book. Because of the mental illness, the claimant must suffer "resulting persistence or marked restriction of daily activities and constriction of interests and deterioration in personal habits and seriously impaired ability to relate to other people." In other words, the impairment reaches a threshold degree when it affects areas in the claimant's life other than work. These criteria, while offering *product* problems of their own, are at least independent of work and therefore do not create the circularity. It is as if the regulations are saying that a mental illness is severe enough if it meets these criteria. But this renders the word *severe* superfluous; one might just as well say (as they do in this section of the regulations) that only mental illnesses with these characteristics count. As a general principle, then, the use of terms of degree, such as *severe*, to qualify mental illness add nothing; at best they are superfluous and at worst they are circular.

As a matter of fact, it is questionable how far these nonwork activities legally can be used as a test of severity. The Court in

Smith v. Califano (1981) stated that disability does not require "vegetat[ing] in a dark room excluded from all forms of human and social activity." It felt that daily activities had limited legal relevance to the ability to work.

Alcohol (and drug) addictions offer special problems. While alcoholism is now generally considered a disease, it is considered to be a self-induced disease. Although evidence shows alcoholism may be inherited, the view prevails that the *tendency* to become an alcoholic is inherited. The people who are more prone to alcoholism should avoid the first drink. The test for determining if a person is an alcoholic is if he or she is "addicted to alcohol and as a consequence has lost voluntary ability to control its use" (*Adams v. Weinberger,* 1977). Even if drinking causes nonemployment, it is considered a *product of mental illness* only if the drinking is involuntary. The symptoms of drinking as a nonaddicted alcoholic and as an addicted alcoholic may be the same—drinking to the extent that one is unable to work—but only the involuntary drinker may be designated sick. Nobody knows how to determine if the drinking is voluntary or involuntary; it is the old familiar determinism-libertarianism dilemma once again. And yet, some doctors believe they can make this distinction. This leads to such philosophically muddled testimony as given by the physician who stated that the alcoholic's condition was not "so deep-seated as to be irremediable," and the "only bar to recovery was claimant's lack of motivation and cooperation" (*Osborne v. Cohen,* 1969).

It is interesting to contrast the acceptance of alcoholism (at least in its addictive form) in the standards of social security disability with its rejection in the standards of the criminal law where the position taken in *Powell v. Texas* (1968) was that the chronic alcoholic should not take the first drink. When compassion is pulling against outrage, society tends to feel that the alcoholic should be held responsible for his or her actions; however, when compassion pulls against indifference, especially in the area where the entitlement is felt to have been earned, society feels that the alcoholic may not have been able to help him or herself. Hence, another general principle emerges: whether a cluster of mental characteristics will be considered to be mental illness may depend on the issue involved and its underlying emotional tensions. One should not expect that mental illness in one area will necessarily be mental illness in another.

Of course, beyond the mental illness and the specific mental characteristics, the standard in social security disability stipulates that the nonemployment be a product of the mental condition. This is the usual *product* dilemma and is encountered throughout this book.

DECIDING THE INDIVIDUAL CASE. The mechanism for determination, review, and steps of appeal of social security disability are described in 20 CFR 404.900. Psychiatrists may have different functions in various levels of this process.

Prior to the determination, information is obtained from treating psychiatrists and other physicians as well as from psychiatric examiners appointed by the social security reviewing agency. Theoretically, at this level the psychiatrist is supposed to give only the medical data. The word *medical* is used liberally throughout the regulations. Stating that one's symptoms (subjective reactions) are not sufficient, 20 CFR 404.1528 adds that psychiatric signs are necessary — "medically demonstrable phenomena which indicate specific abnormalities of behavior, affect, thought, memory, orientation and contact with reality. They must be shown by observable facts that can be medically described and evaluated." Where laboratory tests such as electroencephalography can be helpful, they are included. All of these observations are within the expertise of the psychiatrists; they know how to elicit and observe them.

The problem, of course, comes in the close calls. When a person has a drinking problem, there is no medical way of telling if he or she could voluntarily refrain from drinking. When a person has psychogenic pain without sufficient organic basis, neither the psychiatrist nor the neurologist nor the orthopedist has any medical test of that pain. The best the psychiatrist can do is to describe what the claimant complains of and to gather reports of behavior that are consistent with the claimed degree of pain. They must take the patient's word or do the detective work necessary to show that he or she is malingering (Chapter Five); such detective work does not require psychiatric expertise. Any physician who states that an individual has less pain (or less anxiety or less depression) than he or she reports is accusing the person of malingering. The requirement that "severe and prolonged pain" be a symptom of "a medically determinable impairment" (20 CFR 404.1529) does not have meaning when psychogenic pain is considered. In the less obvious cases, then, where psychiatric expertise is needed most, it may be least applicable.

Fortunately, at this level, the psychiatrist is requested not to make the *product* decision of whether the impairment prevents the claimant from working. This decision is made by the physician, often a psychiatrist, who works in the agency office and makes the initial disability determination from all the reports presented. Social security disability personnel call this a medical determination, although this book assumes that no *product of mental illness* decision is medical. Mental illness evaluations are different from cardiac evaluations. A cardiac disability is exertional and a person with severe heart failure has a medically determinable capacity to expend energy. Trying to distinguish which schizophrenic people cannot work and which will not work (or which alcoholics cannot stop drinking and which will not, or which anxious people with dependent personalities could work if only they wanted to) runs into all the problems discussed in Chapter Three. It really is a societal decision. Given the condition of the claimant, the question is, "Is this the kind of person society feels should be exempt from working and eligible for payment?" To call this decision a medical one is to make the rhetorical error to be described in Chapter Eleven. Just because a doctor makes the decision does not mean that the decision, itself, is medical.

There is no problem with a psychiatrist's making the disability determination; he or she can evaluate the medical reports and, as a member of society, can make the necessary transduction. Instead, a method whereby the psychiatrist was limited to diagnosis and description of signs and symptoms consistent with the diagnosis would be more preferable. The transduction would better be left to a more representative societal decisionmaker and an occupational expert.

When the disability determination has been made, it may be appealed to an administrative hearing and subsequently to the courts. At these stages, the ultimate transductions are made by judges. This is a two-transduction procedure because the judge already has available the disability determination made by the physician at the lower level.

There is an interesting pattern that can be observed, especially with the close calls. Treating psychiatrists are more prone to see the impairment as causing nonemployability; disability determination psychiatrists are less prone to view the nonemployment as a *product of mental illness,* probably because their emotional stance is influenced by a larger view of the needs of the agency. Higher courts, less influenced by agency needs, have had a tendency to overrule agency decisions (Liebman, 1976).

Before leaving this section on social security disability, four general principles will be reviewed.

1. In any standard, the use of terms of degree, such as *severe, substantial,* or *serious,* to describe a mental illness is at best superfluous and at worst circular.
2. Whether a cluster of mental characteristics will be considered to be mental illness may depend on the issue involved and its underlying emotional tensions. One should not expect that mental illness in one area necessarily will be mental illness in another area.
3. Psychogenic pain, suffering, anxiety, and milder degrees of depression are not *medically* determinable.
4. Any doctor who states that an individual has less pain, anxiety, or depression than he or she reports is accusing that person of malingering.

Personal Injury

COMPETING SOCIETAL INTERESTS. Although the law of torts is quite complicated, for these purposes it is sufficient to consider a simple formula: Party A, either by an action or omission of something he or she should have done, causes injury to Party B, for which Party B demands compensation. The competing interests are quite straightforward. Party A (the individual or the insurance company covering the individual) wants to pay as little as possible while Party B (the plaintiff) wants to collect as much as possible.

If the claimed injury is mental illness—often pain and suffering, psychogenic pain, conversion, adjustment disorder, posttraumatic stress disorder (anxiety and personality changes resulting from a massive stress), or postconcussive syndrome (personality changes that may persist long after the physical effects of head injury have disappeared)—psychiatrists may be called upon to speak to two issues. The first is whether the mental illness was caused by the act or omission of Party A. This is not a *product of mental illness* issue. Although it is often a difficult determination to make, it lies within the deterministic framework and thus falls appropriately within the expertise of the psychiatrist. This issue will not be considered here. The second issue is that of the severity of the mental illness. This issue will help determine how much the plaintiff will be compensated. In many cases, the severity is measured by how many former activities the plaintiff is now unable to do. These inabilities become *product* issues in the same manner as was described for social security disability. Ultimately, the decision maker will decide in favor of the plaintiff and will fix the amount of compensation on the basis of compassion—indifference. After listening to the evidence, a compassionate jury will award higher compensation while an indifferent jury will not.

STANDARDS. There are no standards for mental illness in personal injury cases. As in the case of social security disability, any psychiatric reaction can count, so long as it has been acquired under the legally proper circumstances. The loss of previous activities because of the mental illness poses the usual *product* dilemma.

DECIDING THE INDIVIDUAL CASE. Because any mental condition is allowable, if the plaintiff complains of any mental characteristics, the psychiatrist must conclude that there is injury unless there is good evidence that the plaintiff is malingering. Beyond that, a diagnosis may be made. With regard to the limitations of previous activities, it is probably best to report them and discuss how they are (or are not) consistent with this type of person with this type of mental complaint. In practice, however, the psychiatrist often is forced to state whether the limitations are a *product of mental illness* because the courts generally work on a two-transduction system.

The Request for Treatment

COMPETING SOCIETAL INTERESTS. This section will consider the situation where an individual claims to be mentally ill and feels entitled to be given treatment by the government. The issues in this area are quite complex, and in order to understand them in terms of the *product* dilemmas, the area must be defined carefully. The various *product* situations encountered thus far have involved an act (or a specific nonact). They have required one transduction to determine if there is mental illness and another transduction to determine if the act has been caused by the illness. When considering the request for treatment, it is the illness, itself, which must be judged. The behaviors that the individual presents are examined and then it is judged if this cluster of characteristics deserves to be designated as a mental illness. No second transduction is necessary. What society judges are the features of the illness, not its consequences. In Chapter Three it was shown that this process is essentially a *product* situation. The questions asked are *sick or malingering?*, *sick or uneducated?*, or *sick or not significantly deviant at all?* Malingering has been considered in Chapter Five. For the purposes of this discussion it shall be assumed that the individual is not malingering.

While the request for treatment may be considered similar to the right to treatment, there are some important differences. When Birnbaum (1960) popularized the concept of the right to treatment, he was referring to the rights of involuntarily committed mental patients. In some situations, this right has been given constitutional standing (*O'Connor v Donaldson*, 1975; *Eckerhart v Hensley*, 1979). Essentially, the concept is that if the government deprives someone of liberty because of mental illness, that person is entitled to the opportunity for treatment in order that he or she may regain his or her liberty. As used here, the request for treatment refers to voluntary rather than involuntary patients; deprivation of liberty is not at issue. In the right to treatment cases, the State initiates the string of events by abridging the immune right of the individual to be left alone; in the request for treatment cases, the individual initiates the action by claiming an entitlement. By the time the committed patient claims a right to treatment, there is no longer a *product* issue; he or she has already been designated mentally ill at the commitment hearing and during the periodic reviews. These issues have been discussed in Chapter Seven. When a person voluntarily requests treatment, there is very much a *product* issue; someone must decide if the person meets the requirements that entitle him or her to whatever treatment the government offers.

The request for treatment and the right to treatment must be differentiated from the right to refuse treatment. The right to refuse treatment is an immune right, and as discussed in Chapter Seven, it is essentially an incompetence issue. The individual wishes to be treated with indifference. The request for treatment and the right to treatment of the committed patient are essentially claims; the individual wishes to be treated compassionately. Incompetence is not at issue. The claim is that the State must offer (not necessarily give) the treatment; the individual, if competent, may still refuse it.

With these distinctions in mind, the request for treatment in two settings will be considered: the confined setting of the prison and the unconfined setting of society at large.

Although prisoners have been incarcerated involuntarily, their situation is different from that of committed mental patients. Since the prisoners' liberty has not been abridged because of mental illness, they cannot claim a right to treatment in order to restore their liberty interests. Since they previously have not been judged mentally ill, none of the *product* issues have been confronted prior to the request for treatment.

The reasons for providing treatment in prisons are different from those relative to mental hospitals. One court declared that "it is but just that the public be required to care for the prisoner, who cannot, by reason of the deprivation of his liberty, care for himself" (*Spicer v. Williamson*, 1926). The Court in *Estelle v. Gamble* (1976) stated that for a prison to ignore an inmate's serious medical illness would be cruel and unusual punishment, a violation of the Eighth Amendment. Opposing these compassionate tendencies are the financial and political forces tilting the balance toward indifference. Economic resources are limited, and increasing the appropriations for more humane handling of prisoners has never had a high political priority.

In society at large, the average citizen is not confined. In theory, at least, he or she is able to fend for him or herself and is not being punished. Therefore, society must look elsewhere for compassionate interests of those who feel that the government should furnish treatment for mentally ill people who request it. The push for services is rooted in historical trends and the temper of the times. According to Mechanic (1980, pp. 73ff.), the large numbers of people who were mentally unfit for military service in World War II sparked a national focus on the plight of the mentally ill. Congress funded the Joint Commission of Mental Illness and Health whose report (Joint Commission, 1961) prompted the government funding of a vast network of communtiy mental health centers. This movement was supported by other aspects of the temper of the times, especially by a feeling of relative economic affluence, therapeutic optimism, and social activism.

The compassionate interests have two intellectual overlays: ethics and needs. The Task Panel on Legal and Ethical Issues (1978), reporting to President Carter's Commission on Mental Health, maintained that government had an ethical duty to provide service to all the mentally ill and that "society may ultimately be measured in a moral sense from the way it treats its most vulnerable and disadvantaged citizens." The Task Panel on the Nature and Scope of the Problem (1978) estimated that 15 percent of the population needs mental health care. Levine and Willner (1976) estimated that in 1974, mental illness cost society almost 20 billion dollars in lost productivity and time spent by others in caring for the mentally ill (exclusive of treatment). On the basis of such considerations, the Task Panel on Community Mental Health Centers Assessment (1978) recommended that "Those services . . . which can legitimately be denominated health-related should be included under Medicare, Medicaid, and, ultimately, under national health insurance." It would be naive to believe that only compassion motivated these recommendations; professional self-interest also played a role in the suggestions that services be expanded. However, the ethical and need considerations do reflect the compassion that society has for its unfortunate citizens.

Counterbalancing the compassionate interests in entitling the

average citizen to receive treatment for mental illness on request
are the interests that support an attitude of indifference toward the
mentally ill. There is no constitutionally based right of citizens to
be provided medical treatment by the government (*Maher v. Roe*,
1977). Even if the government chooses to provide some services, it
is not obligated to provide all services (*Dandridge v. Williams*, 1970).
As discussed earlier in this chapter, work, independence, and
caring for one's own needs are highly valued in society. Financial
resources are not unlimited. In 1974, direct care of the mentally
ill cost $14.5 billion (Levine and Willner, 1976). As Mechanic
(1980, p. 34) has noted, the expansion of offered services in-
vites increased demand for service; "infinite amounts of money,
personnel, and time could theoretically be absorbed in providing
mental health care." Furthermore, medicine has traditionally been
an independent profession, resisting government intrusion and
regulation. Doctors and hospitals have been wary of service plans
that might curtail their ability to act independently. In addition,
government funded treatment for the mentally ill could provide
economic competition to the private practice of medicine.

STANDARDS. In the prison situation, all persons must be treated
similarly provided they have a requisite mental illness. What
constitutes a serious mental illness, however, has never been made
clear. Once again, a term of degree that adds little clarity surfaces.
The illness must be "medically necessary" and not merely desirable or helpful (*Bowring v. Godwin*, 1977). In practice, in many
prisons serious illnesses are considered to be those with self-
directed violence, extreme depression and bizarre behavior (Gobert
and Cohen, 1981, p. 339).

In society at large, the tilt of the balance between compassion
and indifference has seesawed with the temper of the times, and
although there has never been universal entitlement to treatment
for mental illness, greater or lesser numbers of people have been
considered entitled to government funded treatment on request
(Mechanic, 1980, pp. 83ff.). At the time of this writing, the tide is
swinging towards indifference and fewer people are qualifying for
government funded treatment on request.

The number and types of people qualifying for voluntary treatment is controlled not only by changes in the standards of what

constitutes a mental illness but also by other variations in the guidelines (see Chapter Four). The flow of patients may be regulated by placing a maximum allowable cost per person on services, by limiting the number of inpatient or outpatient visits, by designating the types of professionals who may or must give services or the types of services that may or must be given or the types of institutions in which they may or must be given. Services may be limited to those whose income is under a certain level or may be given only to those who pay something themselves (copayment). None of these guidelines pose *product* dilemmas. Many of them appear in the regulations of Medicare, Medicaid, and rules for mental health centers.

With regard to government funded services to the mentally ill, there has been no attempt to set standards of mental illness as the term is used in this book. The Joint Commission (1961) report included the gamut from "troubled people" to the acutely and chronically psychotic people. The Task Panel on the Nature and Scope of the Problem (1978) included depression, anxiety, insomnia, loneliness, and "other indications of emotional disorders." Even transexual surgery has been deemed medically necessary and therefore covered by Medicaid (*Pinneke v. Preisser,* 1980). As in the case of personal injury, the standard seems wide open. And, as discussed in Chapter Two, using the word *medical* does not add anything to the boundaries of mental illness because the deterministic underpinning of designated illnesses is ultimately not a medical determination. Indeed, what is properly mental illness and therefore properly psychiatric (as contrasted, for example, with non-medical social work) poses its own *product* problems, which will be discussed in Chapter Eleven.

Expanding on some suggestions made by Mechanic (1980, pp. 35ff.) four ways of setting standards of mental illness will be considered, which might qualify for entitlement to government funded treatment. (1) Those conditions would be treated that will produce the greatest gains to society. If psychiatrists had the research data, they could predict which people with which diagnostic categories, when treated, will be most productive. Of course, in such a plan, geriatric illnesses would have a low priority because of the limited life expectancy. Manic people would take precedence over people with schizophrenia because the latter, even when treated, often have a chronic course with residual limitations. And the whole scheme is predicated on the concept that professionals could develop reasonable gain predictions. (2) Those conditions that are treatable would qualify. This is similar to plan 1, but it is without the economic aspect. The problem of defining the nature and efficiency of treatment would need to be resolved. (3) Only the clearly sick would qualify. This is similar to the concept of "sufficient mental illness." Certain diagnostic categories would be chosen by policymakers to qualify. (4) The standards could be left wide open. The first three plans would completely solve the *product* problem, although plans 1 and 2 contain other problems. With designated diagnoses that society's policymakers wish to include in the circle of qualifiers, no further transductions need be performed. The situation here is different from those described earlier in this book where the decision maker would still need to decide if a particular act or nonact were a product of the designated illness. As noted in the beginning of this section, when the behavior under scrutiny is the mental illness itself, only one transduction is necessary—that of judging which clusters of characteristics qualify as mental illness. The fourth plan, that of leaving the standards wide open, shifts this transduction from society's policymakers to the individual decision maker.

What is the role of psychiatric experts in setting up standards in this area? Cameron (1969) echoed the concern of many in the aftermath of the first right to treatment case when he decried the interference of nonmedical judgement in medical matters. However, it has been maintained consistently throughout this book that *product* issues are primarily societal rather than medical matters. The role of psychiatrists is to give information, particularly with regard to plans 1 and 2 to state just what is known and what is not known about the course and treatability of various mental illnesses. Issues concerning the delivery of services may also be discussed. Then it is up to society's policymakers to weigh the balance of compassion and indifference and to determine which diagnostic categories will be included in the standards, or if they will be left wide open.

DECIDING THE INDIVIDUAL CASE. If the standards specify diagnostic categories that are designated as sufficient mental illnesses, the individual decisionmaker has no *product* decision to make. The psychiatrist must make the diagnosis and see if it is on the list. As previously noted, since this area deals with the mental illness itself, no second transduction relating behavior to illness must be made. What is needed is some system of accountability and review to insure that the diagnoses are made accurately and honestly, but this is not a *product* issue.

When the standards are wide open, it is the psychiatrist (or other treatment provider) who makes the decision, as if the decision to designate a cluster of characteristics for mental illness were a medical decision. Florida's mental health laws are typical. Although all people are entitled to voluntary treatment (Fla. S. A. 394.459 [2]), the provision of treatment is subject to the discretion of doctors (Fla. S.A. 394.460) and hospitals (Fla. S.A. 394.465 [1]). From one point of view, this system is not logical, because medical personnel have their own biases when making societal decisions. However, this arrangement does make sense from another point of view. A psychiatrist should not be forced to take on a patient he or she does not know how to treat. When a doctor feels that a patient is not mentally ill, the chances are high that he or she does not know how or does not have the talent to help that person effectively. In addition, the physician's own negative attitudes toward the patient whom he feels is not sick are likely to get in the way. This problem arises in the context of the *product* dilemmas about the scope of our profession, itself. This area will be considered further in Chapter Eleven.

Because of these practical treatment considerations, it seems that the decision to honor the claimant's request for treatment must lie with the practitioner. In actuality, if one practitioner decides not to treat because the individual is not mentally ill, another practitioner usually can be found to take the patient so long as funding is forthcoming. Thus, when the standard is wide open, the *product* dilemma must be decided on the basis of the biases and preferences of the psychiatrist. And the standards that any psychiatrist uses will in no way limit or regulate the number and variety of people eligible for service on request. This limitation can come only from the other types of guidelines enumerated in the section on standards—guidelines which, while responsive to compassion—indifference, do not involve *product* dilemmas in the decision process.

CHAPTER NINE

COMPASSION—INDIFFERENCE
Less Coercive Situations

T he position taken in this book is that the decision of whether behavior is a *product of mental illness* is not a matter of scientific expertise but a matter of social policy. In virtually all the situations considered so far, once the *product* decision has been made by society's representatives, certain consequences inevitably occur. A person designated sick rather than criminal is forced into a mental hospital. The individual judged incompetent to make decisions has those decisions made for him or her by somebody else. The person whose nonworking behavior is adjudicated to be a *product of mental illness* will be entitled to social security disability. The course of action that is followed is taken regardless of the wishes of those whose side in the dispute did not prevail.

There are other *product* situations in which the judgement of illness or nonillness may, but does not necessarily, produce an inevitable result. These are the less coercive situations, and in order to understand them the concept of coercion must be considered first.

Coercion must be distinguished from compulsion. Following Macklin (1982, pp. 25ff.), *coercion* refers to forces brought to bear on the individual from the outside; *compulsion* refers to forces from within the individual that affect his or her behavior.

Whenever forces are regarded, the dilemma of determinism versus libertarianism appears. "What is meant by coercion?" the libertarian might ask. "Doesn't the person have a mind of his or her own? Why couldn't the person choose to resist the outside pressures?" Or, more philosophically perplexing, "How do we know the person was forced to do such and such by outside pressures?

Perhaps the person chose the particular course of action."

When malingering (Chapter Five) was considered, a similar problem was confronted. It had to be decided whether the symptoms that were exhibited were compelled or chosen (consciously simulated). The philosophical problem was resolved by shifting the criterion to whether the symptoms *felt* compelled or chosen and some of the methods by which psychiatrists might infer what the individual was feeling were described. Now, in the case of outside forces, the issue for the libertarian is coercion on the one hand versus the choice or compulsion on the other. The issue for the determinist is coercion versus compulsion. Once again, the philosophical dilemma can be avoided by shifting the criterion. Coercion exists when the individual *feels* that he or she is being forced or changed from without; compulsion or choice exists when the person *feels* forced or changed from within. However, in addition, coercion requires that there is in actuality a relationship regarding the behavior in question between the person and those who he or she feels are coercing. The paranoid schizophrenic person who feels his or her movements are controlled by sinister persons whom he or she has not met is subject to compulsion rather than coercion.

Of course, this is not an either-or situation. There might be both compulsion or choice from within and coercion from without. Therefore psychiatrists should refer to degrees of coercion. The stronger the coercion, the more the individual feels that his or her own wishes or impulses are abrogated by outside pressures. Weakly coercive inputs from without may still exert pressure, but the individual feels better able to resist them.

There are two ways to detect coercion when it is defined as a feeling of outside pressure. The first method is to ask the person how he or she feels, what he or she wished to do, etc. Then, the outside sources can be questioned about what they are trying to accomplish with the individual. Inputs that are in conflict with what the individual wishes are coercive, although they may be so weakly coercive that the coercive aspect is of no practical consequence. The more the person feels forced by the input, the greater the degree of coercion. The second method of gauging coercion has been suggested by London (1969, pp. 28ff.). The greater the degree of coercion by influences without, the more highly predictable will be the consequences of those influences.

A rough scale of degrees of coercion can be constructed. Consequences of legal decisions such as those described in the previous chapters are very highly coercive. When the State has decided that an individual will be committed to a mental hospital, his or her entering the hospital is a highly predictable fact and the person feels that his or her wishes are being abrogated by powerful outside forces. Direct bodily manipulation and the use of certain drugs are highly coercive. Threats, while somewhat less coercive, still have substantial influencing power. Manipulation, which goes on without the individual's being aware of being deceived by the influencer (Bursten, 1973a, Chapter 1), is probably more coercive than persuasion. Even psychotherapy and education, as London pointed out, are somewhat coercive, although the fact that their results may be quite unpredictable and the individual may not feel that his or her wishes are strongly overridden make them relatively weak coercive measures.

This chapter, then, will deal with some situations in which the decision to designate behavior as sick leads to less coercive consequences than the situations previously described. Issues in psychotherapy, social advocacy, milieu therapy in the mental hospital, and the unfit parental relationship will be considered. Simply put, society seems to have less interest in the *product* questions involved in these situations, and therefore, the full legal power of society is not pressed to enforce the consequences of the decision. Why should that be? What about these situations is so different from the others that society is less involved and does not lend its coercive weight?

In Chapter Two, six criteria of illness were described: (a) a cluster of characteristics which is (b) undesirable, (c) natural and rationally explainable, (d) predominately biological, (e) individual rather than social, and (f) beyond the individual's control or choice. While there must be general agreement about all of these criteria in order for illness to be designated, in the situations described thus far, the emphasis has been on the crippling of the choosing mechanism with a resultant loss of the ability to control. There has been general societal agreement that the behavior in question in undesirable (sick, criminal, unwise, manipulative, lazy, etc.), and the *product* debate focused on whether the person could help him or herself. Society, of course, takes a strong interest in behavior, which most everyone thinks is undesirable, and it follows that society would have regulations governing what happens to the person when the *sick or* _____? question has been decided.

In the situations to be considered in the present chapter, however, there is not general agreement about the undesirability of the behavior in question. The focus of the *product* disagreement is on that criterion rather than on the question of choosing. And even when most people might agree that the behavior in question is undesirable, it is not seen as so highly undesirable that society *must* do something about it. Particularly in a society such as in America where the right to be left alone is a fundamental value and encouragement is given to the widest variety of expressive behaviors, society is not prone to intervene unless there is a rather general consensus that the behavior in question is significantly undesirable.

As the focus shifts from control to undesirability, so does the nature of the transduction. Decisions in this area do not center around transductions from determinism to libertarianism; they hinge on the tranduction from fact to value. Instead of asking, "Is this the kind of person who society feels should be able to control him or herself," the transducer must ask, "Is this the kind of behavior that society feels is undesirable?"

With the focus of the *product* question on undesirability of the behavior rather than on choice and control, the issue of competing value systems appears more prominently. When psychiatrists term behavior sick they are saying that it is not good and should be changed. The individual in question may disagree. In the areas considered in this chapter, since society in general does not have a concensus about whether the behavior is highly undesirable, it does not become involved in this conflict in values provided there are no gross improprieties in the actions of either party. Any coercion on the part of the doctor must be less forceful than in the situations backed up by a societal consensus.

If the *product* situations to be discussed in this chapter arise when the psychiatrist feels certain behavior is undesirable while the individual in question and others do not feel it is so bad, is it possible that when psychiatrists make decisions predicated on the notion that someone is mentally ill, they are purveying ideology and values as well as medical treatment? This is not a new charge; Szasz (1970) made it throughout the 1960s. Marcuse (1964) attempted to show that much of what psychiatry regarded as normal (not sick) behavior was geared to maintain the political and economic status quo of the dominant American society. More recently, Robitscher (1980, Chapter 20) has echoed the charge.

Are psychiatric decisions value laden? Of course they are. If sickness is a matter of policy, decisions based on the sickness concept *must* be value laden. Beyond that, any purveyor of anything in society is also to some degree a purveyor of values. People are all children of their cultures and therefore regardless of whoever they serve, they are agents of society as well. And further, any discipline such as psychiatry, which deals with human behavior, is particularly prone to deal with values. There is no getting away from it.

Therefore the substance of these writers' charge is correct, but the charge, itself, is misguided. The detractors of psychiatry are stating a fact, not a charge; there is nothing inherently wrong with making value-laden decisions. If there were, everyone would have to close down shop — including those who level the charge, for in doing so they purvey their own values. The charge is an *ad hominem* rhetorical device used to befuddle the issue when the accuser's values differ from the predominant psychiatric ones.

The problem is not that values are purveyed; the problem arises when, in the course of professional activities, people attempt to impose their values on an unwilling or unsuspecting individual. This can occur in two ways: they may pass off their value judgements as scientific expertise (the subject of this book), and they may use their status in society as experts to coerce others to do what they do not wish to do. The solution, of course, is to be as little coercive as possible.

To review the discussion thus far: the *product* situations to be presented in the present chapter have less coercive consequences than those encountered previously. Society is less apt to lend its weight to these kinds of decisions because there is less societal concensus about the undesirability of the behavior in question. The *product* disagreement is focussed on value conflicts about which society does not take a strong position. The attempt to impose values is an inevitable aspect of the psychiatric enterprise and therefore, the least possible coercive techniques should be employed.

Because society tends not to become involved in the kinds of situations under consideration, modifications must be made in the three stage decision analysis proposed in Chapter Four. In these situations, the competing interests may not be *competing societal interests*. The competition is often on a much more restricted level—between the psychiatrist and the individual in question. The competing interests are competing value systems that lead the doctor to label certain behavior as significantly undesirable and the other person to state that it is not undesirable. There are no standards set up by society's policymakers because, as a reflection of the underlying philosophy of allowing a wide diversity of views and values, society does not become involved. Therefore, there is no template to which a decision maker can fit the facts and opinions when deciding the individual case. Each participant is on his or her own; the matter will probably be decided (one or the other value will prevail) at least partly on the basis of how much coercion the doctor is able to apply to the individual in question.

PSYCHOTHERAPY

There is a wide variety of psychotherapies, and the imposition of the therapist's values on the patient may occur in all of them (London, 1969, pp. 48ff.; Karasu, 1980). Psychoanalytic psychotherapeutic orientation will be used to illustrate some of the *product* dilemmas therapists and patients encounter. Ways of attempting to cope with these dilemmas will also be presented.

While the degree of coercion in psychotherapy is substantially less than that exerted by judicial decisions, it can be significant. In general, the coercion derives from the relative positions of doctor and patient. The patient comes seeking help from a person whom he or she feels has certain technical skills. To a certain extent, the patient feels he or she needs to be in treatment and may be willing to put up with quite a bit because of that need.

Even if the doctor were to disclaim any special knowledge or skills, the patient would likely feel that this disclaimer is part of the technique (as indeed it may be). There is a built-in belief that the psychiatrist's opinion is probably worth more than the patient's. The expectation that the psychotherapist can help is, itself, therapeutic (Frank, 1971); however, it does predispose the patient to trust the inputs from without a bit more than those from within.

As the therapy procedes, the patient develops transference. Essentially, this is a process wherein the patient relates to the therapist in a manner similar to the relationship with his or her parents as he or she was growing up. This, too, is an important and valuable development during the course of psychotherapy, but it further fortifies the feeling of having to do the psychiatrist's bidding and being fearful of disagreeing with the therapist. Identification with the therapist is common and may lead the patient to replace his or her own values with those assimilated from the psychiatrist (London, 1969, pp. 55ff.).

From the standpoint of the psychotherapist, the tendency to coerce, however harshly or gently, stems from what Balint (1964, Chapters 16 and 17) referred to as the "apostolic function." He wrote (p. 216), "[E]very doctor has a vague, but almost unshakably firm, idea of how a patient ought to behave when ill...*It was almost as if every doctor had revealed knowledge of what was right and what was wrong for patients to expect and endure, and further, as if he had a sacred duty to convert to his faith all the ignorant and unbelieving among his patients*" (Balint's italics). It is doubtful whether any psychotherapist—medical or nonmedical—ever entirely relinquishes this feeling.

These, then, are some of the coercive elements in the psychotherapeutic relationship. An examination of how they apply to the disposition of product dilemmas that may arise during psychotherapy follows.

Whom Do We Take Into Treatment?

Several years ago, a young college student was referred for psychoanalysis. He had recently come to the realization that he was sexually attracted to men rather than to women. On a trip home, he announced to his father that he was homosexual. The father responded by promising that he would get his son the "best medical treatment available." The young man related his story to a psychiatrist and inquired whether he could be cured of his homosexuality. After the student gave a detailed history, he was asked if he was uncomfortable with his homosexuality. While he was uncomfortable with his father's reaction and he knew that life as a homosexual man had its special problems, attraction to men felt perfectly natural to him. He did not see homosexuality as inherently undesirable. If an attempt to cure him were made, his sexual orientation would be branded by the psychiatrist as an illness (undesirable). The student probably would have accepted the doctor's recommendation just as he had followed his father's prescription. Is same-sex attraction an illness; are homosexual life-styles *products of mental illness?*

The young man discussed his dilemma with the psychiatrist, and they concluded that his homosexuality either could be considered or could not be considered a disease. It depended on what felt right to him. After a few sessions, during which he discussed the stressful interaction with his father, the young man decided he was comfortable with his life-style, and hence he did not need treatment.

In general, if the patient does not feel that his or her presenting complaint is undesirable, optional ways of looking at it and what treatment methods might be available if the patient were to decide that he or she wants help should be outlined. Halleck (1971) proposes that informing the patient and spelling out options is a good antidote to coercion. It usually is not necessary to make dire predictions: "If you don't come into treatment, such and such will happen." Often, the accuracy of dire predictions are overvalued. However, the person should be invited to come back or to call the psychiatrist at any time in the future if he or she has things that need to be discussed.

There are exceptions to this procedure, of course. In the discussion of undesirability in Chapter Two, it was noted that some clusters of characteristics generally are considered so undesirable that unequivocally it can be said that the criterion of illness is met. For example, a young woman was brought to a psychiatrist by her mother. A schoolteacher, she recently had lost control of her classroom because she could not keep her speech on a single track.

She was so distractable that she would leave the classroom. Attendance at work had become very spotty. Her house was a mess, her mode of dress was becoming more and more outlandish, and she had been up the entire previous night doing such activities as painting her windows with jelly.

This woman showed all the stigmata of mania during the evaluation. However, she did not feel that her behavior was undesirable; indeed, she had experienced a new freedom in living and was enjoying it. The psychiatrist disagreed and firmly told her she was sick and should be in the hospital. She was agreeable to his recommendation and responded very well to a brief hospitalization and treatment with lithium carbonate.

How Much Should Be Treated?

The amount of treatment to be given raises issues that are similar to those discussed in the previous section. For example, a patient, a man in his late twenties, had just suffered the loss of his girl friend. She had left because she felt that he was not contributing enough to the relationship. She had to make all the plans and decisions. When they had first met, she had misinterpreted his inability to be decisive as a kind of sharing and fairness; he would respect her by not dominating her. However, as his respect was revealed to be dependency, she pulled back and ultimately left. This was not the first time this theme had emerged in the patient's life. He complained that he always made a good first impression, but then something seemed to go wrong. His employment record also showed telltale signs. He was in a business field, and because he was bright and well trained, he had little trouble in being employed. As he would begin to advance up the ladder, however, he would become troubled by the increasing independence and responsibility. He had been laid off one job for inadequate performance; he had quit two others because he did not like the work as he advanced. This man was in an awkward employment position; he was too well trained and too bright to stay down at a level in which temperamentally he would have been more comfortable.

This story was not what made him seek help. His complaint was of depression—sad mood, listlessness, preoccupation with the lost girl friend, fitful sleep, loss of taste for food, etc. As he talked, his face was downcast and he sighed. He said that he did not know what to do and he asked for help.

The separation had taken place one week earlier, and already the depression had lifted a bit. Talking with a psychiatrist seemed to help. He was diagnosed as suffering from an adjustment disorder with depressed mood and either dependent or histrionic personality disorder. He complained about the first but not the second condition.

The diagnosis of the adjustment disorder did not pose a practical *product* dilemma. Both the patient and the psychiatrist agreed tacitly that the condition was undesirable and met the other illness criteria. He was willing to be helped and, depending on the degree of professional expertise, he could be helped.

However, the diagnosis of personality disorder posed significant *product* problems. The psychiatrist detected a repetitive pattern, a destructive thread that ran through this man's life. Even the manner in which he related in therapy reflected his reluctance to take on responsibility. But, as questioned in Chapter Two, are personality disorders illnesses? It could be called a *disorder* or even a *problem* but the dilemma would be the same, because the issue was not what it was called but whether it reached a high enough threshold of undesirability to invoke treatment. The stakes were reasonably high, because while his depressed mood would lift within a week or two, a therapeutic attempt to alter his personality style could be long and costly.

The world is full of dependent and histrionic people, and while their conditions may cause problems for them, they neither seek nor want treatment. They do not see themselves as falling within the circle of people called mentally ill. They generally want to be left alone (treated with indifference)—except in crises—and they tend to attribute their difficulties to the actions of others. And, as previously noted, society has neither set up standards for this situation (drawn a circle of illness) nor will it provide an arbitrator to make the decision.

A good case could be made for viewing the patient's personality disorder as illness. It seemed doubly undesirable, not only because it interfered with his optimal functioning but because it contributed to situations that brought on the other illness—adjustment disorder with depressed mood. A compassionate doctor cannot ignore such conditions. Here is the junction at which the *product* decision and the degree of coercion become tied together. With what force, with how much zeal should the patient be convinced that he has a second illness which should be treated? (And particularly this patient, with his propensity for relying on others to make his decisions anyhow!) If he wants to stop treatment when his depression has lifted, should he be told he still needs more treatment? If he declines, should another *product* decision be made and should his refusal to continue be interpreted as a sign of his pathology — a psychological defense against the anxiety of finding out why he has so unproductive a pattern?

There are no easy answers to these questions. A physician has the duty to inform the patient of the findings. The man had a right to a professional opinion, even if in part it were based on compassion. As such, the observations and the data on which the diagnosis was made was outlined for the patient. By pointing out the repeated pattern and raising the possibility that this behavior might reoccur in the future, the psychiatrist was within scientific expertise. However, describing the personality disorder unavoidably also told the patient he was sick and could be treated for an illness. Therefore, this discussion was followed up by telling the patient that he was the one who would have to decide how uncomfortable this pattern made him (essentially, how undesirable he felt it was). He would have to balance the degree of discomfort against the emotional and financial costs of treatment. In other words, the psychiatrist attempted to reduce the impact of the transduction by invoking the concept of *sufficient mental illness* (Chapter Four). The patient would make the ultimate decision; even if the personality style were designated as an illness, did he have sufficient mental illness to fall within the circle of those who must be treated?

In these situations, then, the psychiatrist must go a bit beyond giving the patient information about the options; he or she should point out explicitly that the ultimate decision about the cost-benefit analysis (sufficient mental illness to invoke treatment) must lie with the patient. This tends to minimize the *product* aspect of the decision and is probably the best way to reduce the degree of coercion in a situation which, by its very nature, is coercive. The patient in the present example decided to stop when his depression lifted.

Acting Out

Once psychotherapy has been underway for a while, both patient and psychiatrist have a larger stake in preserving the integrity of the treatment. The patient has already decided that there is sufficient illness to merit treatment and he or she relies on the therapist to keep the enterprise going even if it hurts. The patient has learned that defenses will be erected to protect him or her from the pain of self-discovery. These defenses may lead the patient to disagree with the therapist's view on one day, only to realize later on that the doctor's view had merit after all and that the disagreement was in the service of avoiding painful thoughts and feelings. This is not to say that the therapist is always right and the patient is always wrong, and that is where the difficulty arises. This problem will be illustrated by discussing acting out.

Although the term *acting out* has been jargonized in the unfortunate manner to be described in the discussion of milieu therapy, its original and precise meaning is behavior in which a patient engages in order to avoid thinking about conflicts within the therapeutic situation (Freud, 1914). For example, a rather non-aggressive man may have harbored considerable anger toward his parents when he was younger. Being afraid of their retaliation, he repressed his feelings and turned into a polite and compliant individual. During the course of his psychotherapy, the earlier anger is stirred, and he gains only the most vague memory of it. Because of the tendency to repeat earlier interactions within the therapeutic situation, the patient feels the faintest stirrings of annoyance toward the therapist.

It so happens that the patient's next door neighbor has been trying to get him to join a protest group which feels that the city administration has been favoring slumlords to the disadvantage of the poor. While in the abstract not unsympathetic to the issue, the patient characteristically did not want to get involved with such an antagonistic group. Now, he begins to find the neighbor's arguments more persuasive. He joins the group and becomes a rather vocal advocate for the tenants. Whatever fleeting glimpses he may have had of his anger toward his parents or his annoyance toward his therapist are now firmly repressed; his attention is fully rivetted on his new-found social activism.

From the standpoint of the therapy this is acting out. It is part of the pathological process and quite undesirable—a *product of mental illness.* From the patient's standpoint, this is a new-found freedom to express himself—if anything, it is praiseworthy rather than sick. Indeed, now he is ready to challenge the doctor on the grounds that the psychiatrist just does not like the patient's politics.

At this point, the strategy of minimal coercion—allowing the patient to decide that the behavior is not sufficient mental illness to bother about—is not practical; the investment in therapy is too high and if the therapist is to keep faith with the patient, he or she must try to get the individual to understand what is happening. Fromm-Reichmann (1950, p. 123) recommended that "the psychiatrist should immediately discourage all acting out processes in the neurotic" because they interfere with the investigative process of therapy. Whether this is always practical or necessary may be subject to some dispute among psychotherapists. However, when the disagreement develops, the psychiatrist must attempt to help the patient understand what the behavior means in terms of the therapy. One possible way of proceeding is to answer the patient's objections with a *perhaps sick* and *praiseworthy* paradigm. This does not mean taking a position on the politics of the situation or on the patient's wish to participate, but whatever else the behavior may represent, it is also resistance—and the analysis of this resistance is the immediate therapeutic task. This is more coercive than the suggestion made in the previous section; there is no way around it. And if the patient continues to focus on the protest movement without simultaneously doing the work of therapy, the psychiatrist must be more coercive yet and raise the question of whether the treatment profitably can continue while the individual is so totally wrapped up in the protest movement.

This course is largely within the area of expertise because the main issue is not what is sick and what is not, but rather what aids and what impedes the course of treatment. However, no therapist focuses on every behavior, and it is entirely possible that the behavior singled out as acting out may be particularly undesirable because of the values held by the practicing psychiatrist. This, then, becomes a *product* issue. When the behavior is discouraged more because of its undesirability than its actual therapeutic effect, the psychiatrist has moved from the area of expertise to the *product* area of opinion. This problem will be discussed further in the next section.

Interpretation

Interpretation, as the term is used here, refers to the comments the therapist makes aimed at showing the patient his or her hidden thoughts and feelings. In this way, the patient may become aware of conflicts that he or she has been keeping out of his or her awareness because they are too uncomfortable to contemplate. Interpretations are not given all at once. It is a slow, painstaking process of uncovering the many disguises that some of the patient's more fundamental problems have assumed. Since it procedes by gradual stages, the differences in values between doctor and patient—the differences in opinion about whether certain thoughts and feelings are sufficiently undesirable to be called sick—may be imperceptible, in contrast to the example presented to illustrate acting out where the differences abruptly are apparent to both parties. While patient and doctor may have agreed at the outset about the thoughts, feelings, and behavior representing sufficient mental illness to need treatment, the road to cure is paved with many other thoughts, feelings, and behaviors that may never be considered as value differences. The therapy inevitably covers much more than originally was contracted for (London, 1969, pp. 52ff.). It is unavoidable that the therapist's personal values as well as the values of his or her professional ideology will influence when and how the interpretation is made. For example, therapy has been accused of favoring moral permissiveness (Robitscher, 1980, p. 400), bias against the aspirations of women (Chessler, 1972), promoting adjustment rather than justified political rebellion (Galper, 1973), trying to define acceptable sexual behavior (Robitscher, 1980, pp. 381ff.), and fostering the notion that most problems stem from within rather than from an inequitable society (Dumont, 1968).

These are *product* issues because, in the interpretation, the patient's views are defined as illness and the emphasis is on the undesirability of his or her values. The interpretations are coercive for all the reasons enumerated at the outset of this chapter, and even more coercive because neither party may realize that values are being transmitted with the expertise. But there is expertise here as well, because experience teaches that this process often does lead to a resolution of the problems for which the patient sought help.

Thus the question arises whether it would be possible to strip away the values that parade as illness and leave only the therapeutic expertise. Psychiatrists do know that it is possible to replace certain values by other ones and still have a successful psychotherapy; not all the particular values transmitted by any therapist are necessary. However, it is not possible to have a therapy with no values whatsoever. As mentioned earlier in this chapter, values are part and parcel of every enterprise and particularly of enterprises involved with human thoughts, feelings, and behavior. The only safeguard, and it is a small one, is for the therapist to be aware of the problem and his or her own biases and to be as open-minded as possible. Halleck (1974) noted that the pace of therapy is sufficiently slow to allow ample time for the patient to evaluate what is going on. Further, it should also allow the therapist ample time to ask whether this or that value is really essential to the process.

This suggestion does not pretend to solve the problem. The paradox of psychiatry is that if professional expertise is used, simultaneously psychiatrists go beyond their expertise. To the degree that the method is that of human interaction, this paradox is inevitable; this can be understood if professionals realize that behind all the intellectual and rational aspects of human interaction lies a bedrock of emotion.

SOCIAL ADVOCACY

In 1960, Hartmann pointed out the danger of psychoanalysis being used to establish a health ethic. He warned that using knowledge to establish a morality based on health and sickness must be avoided—essentially the *product* dilemma. Despite this warning, psychiatric values have so permeated the overall societal viewpoint that Lasch (1976) compared psychiatrists to priests: "Just as priests once defined good and evil for the rest of the community, psychiatrists now explain the difference between mental sickness and health ... they pronounce, like priests, on both moral and philosophical questions ... [in] the search not for glory or salvation, but for a sense of personal well being." Robitscher (1980, Chapters 19 and 20) has discussed the extent to which psychiatric values have filtered into society. Whether advocacy of health values is a proper role for psychiatrists is a matter for debate, but such advocacy is inevitable and unavoidable. The public reads the books written by psychiatrists and the media listens to the papers presented at conferences. The field of psychiatry is of great concern and interest, and, as discussed in the previous section, the teaching and practice of this area of expertise automatically transmits values that go beyond expertise. Professionals do become social advocates by implying the degree of undesirability of thoughts, feelings, and behaviors that is sufficient to be called illness; the only real subject for debate is that of how vigorous psychiatrists should be in social advocacy.

A way of mitigating, although not obliterating, this effect has been suggested in the previous chapters and can be generalized here. Advocacy, itself, is less coercive than the force of law. The policymakers or society at large may either listen to or repudiate psychiatrists. However, psychiatrists may be advocates in coercive situations, such as advising the legislature how to set up commitments laws, or in less coercive situations, such as lecturing parents on the dangers of teenage sexual activity. In the discussion of the more coercive situations, it was suggested that setting up standards of sufficient mental illness and sufficient specific mental characteristics to trigger decisions was a matter for society's policymakers, not for psychiatrists. Psychiatrists could stay reasonably within their expertise by describing various syndromes. The policymakers could then make the transduction; they could decide if these clusters of mental characteristics describe persons whom they thought should have the ability to choose and to control themselves.

As noted earlier in this chapter, in the less coercive situations, the emphasis shifts from the choosing criterion of illness to the undesirability criterion. In these areas, advocacy in terms of which behavior is a product of health and which is a product of illness usually speaks to the desirability of the behavior. If it is said that masturbation is not a feature of poor mental health, a transduction is being made. It is inferred that people with this characteristic are the kind of people society generally feels do not have undesirable traits. This type of transduction can be avoided by speaking in terms of predictability rather than in terms of health: Masturbation does not lead to insanity, blindness, sex crimes, acne, or loss of power (sexual or otherwise). All this is within the area of expertise, based on the factual mode of science. The listener can make his or her own transduction into values. Some might say, "OK. Then it's not unhealthy (not undesirable) because it does not lead to these undesirable consequences." Others might disagree: "Even though it does not cause all these bad consequences, it is sufficiently undesirable in its own right to be called sick."

One advantage of avoiding the health transduction is that it tends to force professionals to ask if they really have sufficient scientific data to offer predictions. It is one thing to say such and such is unhealthy; it is quite another to say such and such leads to so and so.

This is not to say that illness should never be implied. It seems perfectly appropriate for psychiatrists to say that lead-based paint is dangerous because some children are likely to eat it and to suffer encephalopathy or disease of the brain as a result. In this case, there is sufficient societal agreement about the undesirability of encephalopathy so that the term *illness* can be used legitimately. However, when it is said that the apathy of the poor who have little economic opportunity is an illness, there are many who would argue that apathy, while undesirable, is not sufficiently undesirable to constitute illness (or sufficient mental illness).

Does that mean that psychiatrists, individually or collectively, should never make moral judgements? Of course not. As citizens, they should speak out. As an organized profession, they may wish to state an opinion. As professionals, they may say that they have seen the distress caused by unwanted pregnancies, and consequently they feel that such distress is sufficiently worth avoiding; therefore, abortion should be legal. Alternatively, they may say that, as professionals, they have seen many women tolerate the distress and adjust to their situations; therefore, they feel the distress is not sufficiently worth avoiding in view of the moral implications. In doing this, they have identified fact as fact and value as value and have not confused the two by using the terms *sickness* and *health.*

Of course this way of advocating will not avoid entirely the *product* dilemma because the public will often hear utterances as the dictum of sickness and health. However, professionals should not take advantage of this fact by going any further beyond their expertise than is necessary.

MILIEU THERAPY IN THE MENTAL HOSPITAL

Putting people in mental hospitals may accomplish two major purposes. In the first place, the individuals are removed from society for their safety or the safety of others or because they are bothersome or because they just cannot cope with living on the outside. In the second place, they are put in the hospital because the institution offers something therapeutic that would not be available elsewhere. Generally, these hospital-specific treatments do not include medications or psychotherapy because these types of treatment could just as well be given on an outpatient basis if safety or bothersomeness were not at issue. Milieu therapy refers to features of the hospital, itself, which either provide something therapeutic or remove the patient from something antitherapeutic in the outside environment.

Although there is some overlap, milieu therapy is conceptually different from treating the patients humanely and with dignity. It is aimed toward treating the individual patient according to his or her needs rather than treating patients as a class (Menninger, 1932). The rationale for humane and dignified treatment is that patients are people and therefore they deserve respect. The rationale for milieu therapy is that patients are sick and need treatment.

The essence of milieu therapy lies in identifying certain behaviors that are *products of mental illness* and bringing the social forces of the hospital to bear on them in order to change them into more healthy patterns. This is often done in conjunction with medication and psychotherapy. The types of interventions that are used will be discussed shortly; first to be considered are the kinds of behaviors that are regarded as sufficiently sick to be targeted for change. Maxmen et al. (1974, p. 36) state that the "therapy sets as its goal the diminution of the patient's specific maladaptive activities and the augmentation of his adaptive behaviors." "Maladaptive" is used synonymously with *sick;* other terms used in the jargon of milieu therapy are *inappropriate behavior* or *acting out behavior,* often not in the context of conflicts stirred up in psychotherapy but in the context of behavior disapproved of by the hospital. In this context, *acting up* is preferred because it has more of a bad than sick connotation and therefore puts more emphasis on the evaluative aspect.

What is the justification for treating maladaptive behavior in a hospital rather than in a prison or reform school — or, for that matter, not treating it at all? The justification, of course, is sickness. In the hospital, the emotional tone is compassion ("This hurts me more than it hurts you, but it is necessary for your mental health!") And often, the patient does not want to be treated with anything but indifference for certain "maladaptive" behaviors.

Patients generally come into mental hospitals one of three ways: They may be committed, in which case there is society's judgement that some of their behaviors are *products of mental illness* as described in Chapter Seven. They may come in voluntarily, in which case the patient and doctor agree that the behavior in question is sufficiently undesirable to qualify as mental illness. Or they may come in under pressure from others despite the fact that they do not see their behavior as sick. There are no further *product* dilemmas once society has stamped certain behaviors as sick nor is there a problem with trying to treat those behaviors that the patient and doctor agree to call ill. However, there may be disagreement between patient and doctor about the appropriateness of behaviors that prompted the hospitalization or behaviors that have been observed since the time of the admission. Any attempt to treat these activities puts the psychiatrist in the position of having decided unilaterally that the behavior is sufficiently undesirable to be called sick — a *product* conclusion beyond expertise.

What types of behavior are being discussed? Certainly most suicidal actions or dangerously aggressive behavior are referred to. Also referred to is bizarre and disruptive behavior, or lack of behavior such as catatonia or mutism or severe lack of eating as in anorexia nervosa. However, as the reports are reviewed of many therapeutic milieu programs, other behaviors are encountered that have been considered sick; the degree of undesirability of some of these behaviors might be subject to some dispute. Here are just a few examples: An apathetic housewife who does not clean her room, do her laundry, or make her bed: (Maxmen et al., 1974, p. 170); apathy and dependency as indicated by little attention to grooming, room cleanliness, or work productivity (Ayllon and Azrin, 1965); lack of work and productivity (Jones, 1953); recreational use of alcohol and drugs when the nonaddicted patient was on pass, and lateness to appointments; being inactive in the ward community, keeping problems to oneself, not taking responsibility for helping others and for the group as a whole (Almond et al., 1968).

Not infrequently hospital staffs demand performance in some of these areas that exceeds their own practices. Are there no nurses who fail to keep their rooms in order or doctors who use recreational drugs? The rationale for targeting these kinds of behaviors for milieu interventions is that while nurses and doctors are not sick, patients are. Even if this is granted, there remains the question of whether these behaviors belong to the sick aspect or the healthy aspect of the individual, a problem of allocation of *product* raised in Chapter Three. And the degree of group involvement described by Almond et al. is particularly interesting because the subordination of individual interest to group interest on the ward is far in excess of that which characterizes the larger American society (Bursten, 1973b). As noted in Chapter Two, some of the targeted behaviors are considered so generally undesirable that they meet the criterion of illness; others, however, are equivocal and force psychiatrists to go beyond their expertise.

Turning from the behaviors targeted as sufficiently undesirable to the interventions of milieu therapy designed to change them, it can be noted there have been a wide variety of milieu therapy programs (Maxmen et al., 1974, Parts 1 and 2; Robbins, 1980). From the standpoint of this book, they shall be clustered according to their relative degrees of coercion.

At a relatively low coercive level are programs that rely on social approval or disapproval. Often, organized groups of patients discuss each others' behavior to provide feedback. Staff may also participate. Shaping is a more subtle type of feedback where appropriate behavior earns positive feedback and "inappropriate" behavior is ignored.

Somewhat more coercive are programs that provide reward (or punishment) systems in order to change targeted behavior. These rewards or punishments are called *reinforcers;* their association with a particular behavior is likely to increase or decrease the patient's use of that behavior. In the token economy, the reinforcers are tokens that may be spent for things or activities the patient likes. Tokens are usually given for specific behaviors. In the step system or ladder milieu, improvements in behavior may be reinforced by "privileges" — increasing ability to have visitors and to move about freely and independently on and ultimately off the unit.

Prescriptive restrictions are even more coercive. Visitation, mail, and telephoning may be cut off if the doctor feels they are medically harmful; even the patient's own clothes may be kept from him or her if a "qualified mental-health professional" feels they are "inappropriate to the treatment regimen" (*Wyatt v Stickney,* 1972). It should not be implied that these prescriptive restrictions are the rule; indeed the law views them as exceptional. However, they are invoked to prevent undesirable behavior and by their nature they are highly coercive.

Many of these interventions are variants of behavior modification techniques, although some are more stringently defined than others. While the potential legality of withholding the reinforcers, which may be visits with staff, recreation, visits outside the hospital, etc., has been questioned, society has generally left their use to the discretion of psychiatrists because they have been seen as in the realm of therapy (Wexler, 1973). But they can only be in the therapeutic realm if the targeted behavior is seen as sick and if the reinforcer changes it in some reasonably lasting fashion. Whether they are necessary for the effective and lasting change of behavior generally agreed to be undesirable is open to question (Bursten and Geach, 1976; Bursten et al., 1980); this is conceivably researchable and thus within the area of expertise. Whether the targeted behaviors are sick is a *product* issue.

It should be apparent that many of the targeted behaviors may represent conflicts of values and that psychiatrists may be on shaky ground when they justify coercive interventions by calling them *products of mental illness.* There are a few measures that can be taken in an attempt to mitigate the situation. (1) They can do more research aimed at identifying just which equivocally undesirable behaviors, when changed, have an impact on the behaviors that both patient (or society, in the case of committed patients) and doctor agree are sick. For example, does coerced good grooming help cure disturbing hallucinations and delusions? (2) They can drop the demands for behavior change where there is disagreement about undesirability if the conditions in the first measure are not met. (3) They can change the term *privileges* to *rights* where the privileges are things enjoyed by most everyone on the outside (Bursten, 1973b). Then, instead of the patients having the burden of earning a privilege by exhibiting good behavior, the staff would have the burden of demonstrating that the targeted behavior was sufficiently sick, and the right must be withheld. This would still leave open the possibility of specific behavioral programs for behavior that both patient and psychiatrist consider sick. (4) When a patient acts up, an earnest attempt is made to discover if the behavior is a feature of mental illness or a response to provocation on the part of staff or patients or to an intolerable ward situation (Bursten, 1973a, Chapter 8). Hospital administrators can monitor units with high incidences of acting up to attempt to minimize provocation of patients.

As in the case of psychotherapy, the hospital milieu will always contain some degree of coercion by which it transmits the values of the staff under the guise of treatment. Social forces can be effective in the treatment of mental illnesses, and once again, in order to utilize expertise, professionals will have to go beyond it to some extent. However, they should try to minimize this process.

THE UNFIT PARENTAL RELATIONSHIP

The issue of the unfit parental relationship arises in child custody disputes. The disputants may be divorcing parents, parents and the State, or parties in a guardianship, adoption, or foster placement proceedings. In some cases, the unfitness of the relationship is undeniable; there is general societal agreement that relationships characterised by parental abandonment, physical injury to the child, incest, etc. are undesirable. These are the "gross failures of parental care" described by Goldstein et al. (1979), and while investigators may be needed to turn up the evidence, no psychiatric expertise is required to tell the courts that such relationships are unhealthy. The situations with which psychiatrists are concerned are those that do not have these gross failures. After attempts at reconciliation, therapy, and mediation have been refused or failed, the psychiatrist may be called in to help the judge make what often is the least noxious decision between the contending parties. As Goldzband (1982, p. 30) noted, such custody decisions require the wisdom of Solomon; it is probably no coincidence that the Bible's first example of Solomon's wisdom was his decision when two women were arguing over the possession of a child — probably the oldest custody dispute on record.

Is the issue of unfit parental relationships in custody disputes properly placed in the present chapter? Are the decisions in these situations less coercive? Is it a matter of the tension between compassion and indifference?

Oster (1965) has discussed the ingredients that go into custody decisions. In addition to the age, sex, health, and preferences of the child, the fitness of the parents is considered. (Although not discussed by Oster, other ingredients include such factors as kinship, race, religion, and even social class.) The Group for the Advancement of Psychiatry (GAP, 1980, Chapter 3) has suggested that professionals focus on the fitness of the relationships rather than of the parents; therefore, the use of the term *parental relationship* emphasizes the impact the parent has on the child.

Oster breaks down parental fitness into moral fitness (which may include misconduct or merely character traits — even political beliefs), love and affection (which is presumed if there are no gross failures of parental care), and the ability to provide for the child physically, financially, and mentally. Of all these factors, it is only in the assessment of the last one—the parental ability to provide for the intellectual and emotional nurturance of the child—that special psychiatric expertise might be required. This may be considered as the fitness of the parental relationship in the narrow sense; this is the aspect of the relationship that is being considered here. And since it is only one of many issues considered by the court, the situation is somewhat different from those discussed in the previous chapters. For example, in the contract nullification situation, the focus of the proceeding is on the *product* question. If signing the contract were a *product of mental illness,* the contract will be nullified; if not, the contract will stand. In the custody hearing, however, even if the parental relationship (in the narrow sense) is found relatively unfit, other ingredients of the decision might outweigh this finding. In the situations discussed previously, the decision turned on the *sick or* _____? question. In the custody situation, the *sick or* _____? question is only one of several questions being asked. In this sense, then, while the custody decision, itself, is highly coercive, the unfit parental relationship aspect of it is somewhat less so.

Compassion—indifference lies at the bottom of the determination of the unfit parental relationship. If the relationship is sufficiently deviant from that which is felt good for the child's development, there is no hesitation to call it sick. In this case, sickness of the parent may be implied by using a diagnostic label or diagnostic-sounding adjectives, such as "the mother is extremely narcissistic." If the relationship is more equivocal, pronouncements may be muted with such terms as *unhealthy* or *unwholesome.* Psychiatric experts characterize the relationships in terms of sickness and health, and prognosticate in terms of the relationship's producing a sick or unhealthy child. All the focus on the child is driven by compassion for him or her. The fitness of the parental relationship hinges on whether compassion should force some intervention or whether the relationships of both disputants with the child are sufficiently adequate that they should not be significant factors in the determination of the issue (treated with indifference).

Because of the complexities of the custody situation, one might still argue whether it is properly placed alongside the other situations described in this chapter. However, there is another reason for doing so. As in the case of psychotherapy, milieu therapy, and social advocacy, the *sick or* _____? judgements made in custody disputes do not focus on the parents' ability to choose or control the nature of the relationships; they focus on the degree of undesirability of the relationships. Values loom prominently in the assessment of unfitness.

Since the ultimate decision is backed up by the coercive weight of society, it should be possible to look at the decision process through the use of the three stages described in Chapter Four.

COMPETING SOCIETAL INTERESTS. As already noted throughout this book, there is a strong basic ideology in the American social and political systems to allow the widest possible diversity. In comparison with many other countries, the American people tend less to prescribe how people should think and act. There is a basic right to be left alone (Chapter Seven). More specifically, the Supreme Court has protected the privacy of the family and the parental right to decide how to bring up children. In *Meyer v Nebraska* (1923), the Supreme Court specifically warned against the State's trying to enforce standards of the ideal child. In *Pierce v Society of Sisters* (1925), the Court insisted that parents have the "liberty to direct the upbringing and education of children under their control." More recently, the Court in *Santosky v Kramer* (1982) stated that the "freedom of personal choice in matters of family life is a fundamental liberty interest ... " This interest "does not evaporate simply because (the parents) have not been model parents."

On the other hand, in its parens patriae role, courts have long been concerned about protecting the interests and welfare of children in custody disputes (*United States v Green*, 1824). As Mlyniec (1977) has observed, the State has swung between minimal involvement in family life and the protection of children from harm. This balance of competing interests is well laid out in *Ginsberg v New York* (1967) in which the Court decided that the State does have an interest in protecting children from obscene reading matter.

STANDARDS. "The prevailing law on child custody mirrors contemporary values shared by the public . . . " (GAP, 1980, p. 21). In a review of these values and their economic and social bases, Roman and Haddad (1978) point out how, during feudal times, woman and children belonged to the Lord of the manor as well as to the husband and father. Subsequently, children were thought to be the property of the father, and it was only during the seventeenth century that the concept that the child was a developing person in his or her own right weakly began to emerge. Partly due to the industrial revolution that tended to cause fathers to spend more time away from home, the pendulum slowly began to swing from the child being the father's property to the child needing the mother's nurturance. The tender years doctrine evolved; young children need their mothers. The prevailing values of motherhood were expressed in rhapsodic tones: "There is but a twilight zone between a mother's love and the atmosphere of heaven . . . " (*Tater v. Tater.* 1938). This presumption that the mother is the more natural parent is still very prevalent. However, it should be noted that the emphasis was not on the child's being the *property* of the mother; the focus had shifted somewhat from property rights to the needs of the child and the parent-child relationship.

Focus on the interests of the child, which had been expressed one hundred years earlier by Judge Story in *United States v. Green* (1824) was stated explicitly and forcefully by Judge Cardozo in *Finlay v. Finlay* (1925), "[The chancellor] acts as parens patriae to do what is best for the interest of the child." "Best interests of the child" has become the predominant standard in many current custody disputes. The problem with it is that it is "weakly defined" (Mlyniec, 1977). Statutes that attempt to define this standard more explicitly invariably end up with a mixture of fact and value criteria. For example, Michigan (C. L. A. ANN., 1971) refers to the stability of the home, the moral fitness of the competing parents, the record of the child in the school and community, the ability of the parents to supply physical needs, etc., all of which may be judged if an investigator can produce the relevant facts; no special expertise is needed, and the judge makes society's value judgements. On the other hand, most prominent in the Michigan criteria of "best interest of the child" is "the love, affection and other emotional ties existing between the competing parties and the child." The relative mental health of the competing parties is also important to the decision. These are the areas where psychiatric expertise is needed, and these are precisely the areas prone to mix fact with values. Except where there is gross parental failure, there is no way to report to the judge without transducing observations (facts) to values. Indeed, even what is choosen to be observed is colored by ideologies and values. The "best interests of the child" standard poses a *product* dilemma in terms of undesirability.

Just which types of parental relationships are significantly undesirable according to society's standards? If this question could be answered, a circle could be drawn around these types of relationships. Those parental relationships falling outside the circle would not be considered relevant to the decision (treated with indifference). The psychiatrist's job, then, would be merely to ascertain whether the relationships are those described within the circle. This would keep them within their expertise.

There is one such circle, but no psychiatric expertise is needed to tell the court if the relationships under scrutiny fit within it: Goldstein et al. (1976) developed standards of gross parental failure, and they can be used to define the circle of sick relationships (unfit in the narrow sense) in custody disputes in general. All other types of parental relationships in the narrow sense are those that ordinarily should not trigger society's intervention in any highly coercive way. Society tolerates strict parents, cold parents, flaky parents, parents who are afraid of their children, mildly retarded parents, etc. All of these should fall outside the circle of relationships which, for purposes of custody determinations, are classed as sick enough to require intervention.

Goldstein et al. applied their criteria of gross failures of parental care only to cases where the State wished to take a child away from its family. These criteria are applied more broadly in this book. One might argue that when the parents are separating anyway and the child must leave one parent, the issue is different; here it must be ascertained which is the *better* of the two parental relationships. However, in custody disputes where subtle rather than gross failures are involved, the facts are so intermingled with values that the State should not consider them.

For example, the following hypothetical case problem can be considered.

Mrs. A. has a borderline personality type. Her thoughts, while not grossly psychotic, are not always too tightly organized. Because she is so unsure of herself, she frequently gives mixed messages to Mary, her daughter. She tends to smother the child to the point where mother and child seem to hold on to each other emotionally for dear life. When Mrs. A. is under stress, she tends to confuse Mary who then feels lost and clings even more closely to her mother.

Because Mrs. A's sense of identity is so ill-formed, she needs someone to lean on. Therefore, she has married a man who is very sure of himself. Mr. A. might be characterized as having a narcissistic personality. He is vain and self-centered and has difficulty in seeing anyone's point of view but his own. In contrast with her relationship with her mother, Mary can be sure of what her father wants from her; he wants her to be a good reflection of him so that he can be proud of her in public.

While a psychiatrist could see problems with both parental relationships, they do not constitute gross failures of parental care; indeed, such types of relationships are not at all rare. The State will not take Mary away from the family even though she is developing the same confused thinking and lack of identity that her mother has. The child's relationship with Mrs. A. is not within the circle of sufficiently ill to necessitate its dissolution, so long as Mrs. A. stays married. If the marriage breaks up (and such marriages often do), the psychiatrist might well find that the child could form a firmer sense of identity under the father's care than with her confusing and smothering mother. When the marriage dissolves, the mother's relationship has moved within the circle. Does society want tacitly to tell borderline women like Mrs. A. that psychiatry (and therefore society) will tolerate their relationships with their children while they are married, but they will lose their children on psychiatric grounds if they divorce? Is the message that if they want to keep their children, they had better remain married?

Of course, if the marriage dissolves and if mediation fails and joint custody is not worked out, one of the parents will lose the child. However, it is questionable whether the decision of who loses should be a psychiatric one. This line of argument can be best developed by dealing with what happens when the individual case is decided.

DECIDING THE INDIVIDUAL CASE. As Beaver (1982) points out, when no gross parental failure has occurred, if psychiatrists attempt to decide which types of relationships are better and which are worse, they are forced to go beyond their expertise in both the predictive and the value respects. They are on very weak ground when they attempt to predict what will happen to the child, because the data observed are often given under stress and duress; they do not know how the relationship may change as the child gets older or when unexpected circumstances may arise; they do not know how much of a desirable feature of the relationship is optimal; and they do not know how much weight they should give to each of the relationship characteristics observed. As Beaver has noted, the ability to predict in this area is not even on as firm a footing as the ability to predict imminent dangerousness in commitment cases.

The second respect in which they must go beyond their expertise is in transducing observations into values and presenting them as expertise; this is the subject of this book. As Beaver states, even if psychiatrists could predict what would happen to the child in the future, "the relative merits of a neurotic over-achiever versus a passive dependent under-achiever (or even a rosy-cheeked regular achiever, I might add) involve issues of philosophy that extend far beyond the professional boundaries of psychology or psychiatry." Values can be easily seen in checklists for the practitioner. Trunnell (1976), for example, proposes an examination to be made of "how in tune with the child is the parent—is the parent 'listening' or 'telling'?" Is the implication that parents should fall within the circle if they believe that children should be seen but not heard because they must learn to respect their elders? And, as so often happens, the checklist even has an item that gauges how flexibly the parents can accept feedback. All too frequently, reports interpret refusal to agree with the psychiatrist as hostility, resistance, and other indicators of diminished capacity to parent.

Another example from a report follows: "Mrs. Anderson has marked emotional immaturity, self-centeredness, and a desire to avoid limits and structure.... Although she would never be negligent or abusive, she does not possess the maturity of judgement to be a well-rounded parent.... She is overly permissive and 'smothering' in her interaction with Betty.... She gave no indication of being able to provide discipline.... She tried to make a good impression ... and she tended to gloss over problems.... Mrs. Anderson will not accept advice which would enable her to change these characteristics." Perhaps Mrs. Anderson and many other mothers like her do not wish to change these characteristics because they feel that little children should be spoiled a bit in order to feel love and have happy dispositions. Should that count against her because the expert says it is immature? Or should it fall outside the circle of intolerable relationships?

Findings in custody evaluations are plagued with the same value problems as are interpretations in psychotherapy. However, there are two important differences. In psychotherapy, the individual has acknowledged sickness and is relying on expertise to help him or her. In the custody situation, the parent has not acknowledged sickness and is entering the psychiatric domain under duress. In addition, psychotherapy is far less coercive; while custody evaluations may or may not be determinative, the ultimate coercive stakes are much higher.

On the basis of these observations, some suggestions have been made regarding participation in custody proceedings in order to minimize going beyond psychiatric expertise. (1) Society should stop looking for the *best* interests of the child. Seeking the *best* leads into subtleties that are too mingled with values. (2) With regard to parental relationships in the narrow sense, society should adopt the view that all such relationships which do not show gross failure reasonably protect the child's interests; they should not fall within the circle of sick (intolerable) relationships. (3) Comparisons between disputants must be made, but since these comparisons are so intertwined with values, they should be made by the judge or by some other representative of society's values. Of course the judge needs help in making these impossible decisions, but psychiatrists should not participate in this process because their facts carry more weight than their expertise warrants. Society should not confuse help with the appearance of help. (4) Participation should be limited either to rebutting the unwarranted testimony of other experts or informing the judge, in the abstract, of the few facts that are known, such as that little children do tend to remember the parents they have left and that they often create unrealistic fantasies about them. Even here ideology must not be confused with fact.

I have discussed these considerations and suggestions with some colleagues—all with experience in the area and people whose opinions are greatly respected. None of them completely agree with what has been stated here. Therefore, these suggestions are offered only tentatively and with some trepidation and hesitation. It may be that the case is overstated. However, the suggestions and the reasoning behind them should be stated and should take their place in the forum of ideas.

CHAPTER TEN

SHAM COMPASSION
Pseudo-*product* Situations

In most of the *product* situations described thus far, some person or group has asked psychiatrists to help in the resolution of *sick or* ____? questions. Whether the inquiry is in the service of the courts as in the insanity defense or the commitment hearing, or in the service of an adjudication board as in the case of social security entitlement, or even in the service of an anxious person privately consulting a psychiatrist, the *sick or* ____? question is central to the decision making of the person or group asking it. These are genuine *product* questions, and those who ask them are genuinely interested in the answers.

However, there are other situations where society or groups within it only appear to be asking *product* questions. Even if the question put to the psychiatrist takes the form of "Is the behavior in question a *product of mental illness?*", there is a very different agenda. The person or group wishes to use the existence or nonexistence of illness as a means to accomplish certain ends that have little to do with illness. Essentially, the *product* information provides it with an excuse. These are the pseudo-*product* situations. In this chapter, situations will be considered such as the decision not to prosecute and disciplinary procedures. The ambiguities of coverage of psychiatric illnesses by third party payers will also be discussed.

In Chapter Four, it was pointed out that all genuine *product* questions are driven by tensions between compassion (on the sick side) and outrage or indifference (on the other side). Compassion is indispensible for a judgement of sickness. By contrast, in these pseudo-*product* situations, those requesting the evaluation are not driven to any great extent by compassion. At best, when sickness will be used as an excuse or rationalization for people to pursue their own ends, the compassion expressed for the individual in question is a sham.

In other words, the pseudo-*product* situations discussed here differ from the genuine *product* situations because of the difference in the emotions and motives of the agency for whom the psychiatrist is working. In these situations, despite the questions the person or group asks, it does not feel compassion, nor does it think the person is really sick. Or, if there is a bit of genuine concern about the health of the individual in question, this concern is far outweighed by other interests of the agency. Whether an evaluation request is a genuine or pseudo-*product* issue depends on whether compassion is one of the strong competing interests behind the request.

No one operates from a position of single and pure motivations. Even in the genuine *product* situations, while compassion is in the forefront, the participants in the drama also have other agendas. Therefore, the difference between the pseudo– and the genuine *product* situations is a matter of degree. The reader will quickly recognize how some of the situations described in the previous chapters shade off into the situations to be considered in this chapter. Indeed, Szasz (1965) feels that all *sick or* _____? decisions are pseudo-*product* situations because whatever compassion there may be is subordinated to the other motives of society's agencies. Many psychiatrists disagree.

If the difference between pseudo– and genuine *product* situations lies in the emotions and motives of those asking the question, how can one know which is which? Sometimes their motives are obvious; sometimes they will acknowledge what their motives are. At other times, their motives can be inferred only by their actions. This is a risky business, and it becomes a matter of judgement. That is why there will not be general agreement about which *product* situations are pseudo and which are genuine. Nonetheless, when the psychiatrist does infer that the compassion is a sham and that the agenda has little to do with the question of sickness, he or she feels used and manipulated. The psychiatrist then usually wants to get out of the evaluations business altogether. However, this option is a luxury that society cannot afford.

THE DECISION NOT TO PROSECUTE

Shoplifting

As indicated in Chapter Six, not all who have committed an offense go through the entire criminal procedure leading up to punishment. The policeman may divert the offender into the mental health system at the outset, and the judge or jury may divert him or her at the time of the trial. Between these two points, there are other opportunities for the offender to be diverted out of the criminal justice system. Much of the power to do this lies with the prosecutor. He or she has considerable discretion about whom to prosecute and whom not to prosecute. Among the facts the prosecutor considers when deciding whether to prosecute are the outrageousness of the crime, the sufficiency of the evidence, the expense of prosecution and the overload of the courts, the existence of alternative methods of incarcerating the suspect, the possibility of unduly harming the suspect, and the anticipated reaction of the community to the decision (Miller, 1969). The charges may be dropped with no consequences or on the understanding that the offender will take some course of action voluntarily, such as psychiatric treatment; or the individual may be required to enter one of several types of diversion programs, such as a drug treatment program (Vorenberg and Vorenberg, 1973).

Not infrequently, psychiatrists get requests from attorneys to evaluate their shoplifter clients. These are usually women. The ostensible reason for the request is that if the prosecutor can be shown that the offense was due to the shoplifter's mental illness, the charges will be dropped. This, of course, would be a rather typical *product* situation. In actuality, however, the compassion expressed for the sick offender is a sham and the procedure is part of a very different agenda. If the offender were brought to trial before a jury, it is unlikely that she would be found not guilty by reason of insanity; her urge to steal is considered to be the kind of behavior that people should control. Indeed, some attempts to plead insanity at a trial have not been successful.

Why, then would a prosecutor take a psychiatric evaluation of such a person seriously? He or she knows it will be ineffective at the trial.

Both defense attorneys and prosecutors have pointed out that shoplifting is not a very outrageous crime and the time and expense of prosecuting in view of the other crimes needing to be dealt with is hardly worth the effort. Often, those sent for evaluation are middle class women who are not the "criminal type"; they come from "good" families and have good reputations in their communities.

If the prosecutor has compassion for the defendant, it is not related to feeling that she is significantly ill; it is related to the fact that "she's not the criminal type of person who should be in jail." This, together with the time and financial costs necessary to carry the case forward will persuade him or her to drop the charges if this is the first or second offense. However, these reasons would not be well received by the community and they are rarely made public. Instead, the prosecutor needs an excuse, and the psychiatric evaluation provides one that will not create waves in the community. For this reason, the request for psychiatric evaluation of shoplifters is a pseudo-*product* situation.

What should be the psychiatrist's response to such a request? Often, the first response is the feeling of being manipulated. Indeed, the psychiatrist who is inexperienced in this area is being fooled because the agenda really is not that of determining if the offender's behavior was *a product of mental illness*. The more experienced psychiatrist realizes what the agenda is, and the attorneys know that the psychiatrist realizes it. There is no need to feel used or manipulated in this situation. Everyone, the defense attorney, prosecutor, and psychiatrist, are involved in a social convention; no one is really being fooled and probably no one is being harmed. It is doubtful that psychiatric treatment is any less effective in dealing with kleptomania than is imprisonment. If there is any harm, it consists in preserving an overburdened court system and the privileges given to "nice" middle-class women. It might be said that psychiatric participation in this convention impedes the necessity of reform (Halleck, 1971, p. 156). Some psychiatrists will feel comfortable as participants while others will not.

While the decision to participate or not may have ethical

overtones, they do not speak to the issues considered in this book. The *product* issue arises only if psychiatrists do the evaluation. And even here, the *product* dilemma can be avoided if the evaluation is handled as a straight clinical matter. A clinical diagnosis can be made; it is usually both kleptomania (which is synonymous with shoplifting) and adjustment disorder. The latter diagnosis is often appropriate because the shoplifting act frequently occurs when the woman is under stress. The woman and the stress she was under can be described. Those making the request usually do not need an opinion about whether the choosing mechanism was crippled by the stress, and this transduction should not be made. Nor should psychiatrists speak to the question of whether the defendant was sufficiently ill to merit exculpation. And certainly, psychiatrists are in no position to state that treatment will cure her; this would be going beyond their expertise in the predictive area.

Thus, for those psychiatrists who wish to participate in this social convention, the evaluation report can be done in such a way that professionals do not go beyond their expertise. The situation is not a genuine *product* situation, nor should it be treated like one.

The Mentally Ill Sex Offender

Among the various methods of diverting offenders out of the criminal justice system are the sexual psychopath laws. While the statues differ among the various states that have them, generally the sexual psychopath (usually a man) is identified as someone who has committed a sex offense (often more than once), who is considered to be a danger to others and to the community, and who cannot control himself/herself because of mental illness (Group for the Advancement of Psychiatry [GAP], 1977). In contrast with many other offenses, in the case of the sexual offense the procedure for this diversion is not the insanity plea. Instead, the offender has a special hearing, which, depending on the state, may be either in lieu of a criminal trial or after he or she has been convicted of the offense. The hearing is considered to be a civil matter, akin to a commitment hearing (*Humphrey v Cady*, 1972). Often, instead of receiving a specific sentence in prison for the offense, the sexual psychopath will be hospitalized for an indeterminate length of time until he or she is deemed cured.

There are several reasons for considering the request for psychiatric evaluation in these cases to be pseudo-*product* questions. While it might be felt that diversion from a punitive environment to a treatment situation expresses the triumph of compassion over outrage as in the case of a successful insanity plea, in practice treatments are not very effective and the offender well may be incarcerated for a much longer time in the hospital. This is especially true for relatively minor offenders (Forst, 1978, p. 47). Indeed, the possibility of keeping the offenders off the streets was a prime reason for the inception of these laws (Brakel and Rock, 1971, p. 341). Kittrie (1971, p. 344) has stated that laws such as those considered in this section merely have been "a pragmatic tool for accomplishing under therapeutic auspices what could not be done at all in the criminal realm." Civil procedure does not require all the safeguards of criminal procedure; it allows indeterminate incarceration, and it allows the punishment (treatment) to be aimed at the kind of person the offender is, rather than at what he or she has done.

Perhaps the best documented explanation of the real use to which sexual psychopath laws are put is presented by Forst (1978, Chapter 3). After studying the views of prosecutors, defense attorneys, judges, and other court personnel, he showed that all parties chose between prison and hospital on the basis of which disposition most likely would result in the longer incarceration. In other words, the laws serve the prosecutor's function of preventive detention (keep the sex offender off the street as long as possible), while the defense attorney attempts to get his or her client out as soon as possible (p. 49).

One further clue that these laws do not serve compassion is the fact that the poor are overrepresented in the long-term hospitalizations for sex offenses (MacNamara and Sagarin, 1977). By contrast, it is the wealthy who have both the means and the desire to plead insanity in other criminal situations.

The sexual psychopath laws, then, provide an alternative form of incarceration. Even if hospitalization produced better results than jail (and that is very doubtful [GAP, 1977, Chapter 5]), it would not mean that evaluating offenders is a genuine *product* task. Many types of interventions might produce certain results without the person ever having been sick. Castration frequently has been recommended as a way of handling sex offenders. It would even have to be done by a doctor in a medical setting. It might even prevent further sex offenses in some people. But all of that does not mean that the individual was sick; it merely means that the individual's behavior was judged highly undesirable and that someone found an effective way to change it. In order to be sick, all the criteria mentioned in Chapter Two must be fulfilled, and in addition, the behavior must evoke the compassion of others.

Thus, in contrast to the insanity defense, the sexual psychopath laws present pseudo-*product* questions. And, it seems that the possibility of doing harm is much greater than in the shoplifting area. Here, there are conflicting parties and a decision is called for. How should the psychiatrist handle the requests for these kinds of evaluations?

In the first place, the usual standards for inclusion in the circle of mentally ill sex offenders are broad and nonspecific. And even though the written standards in the insanity defense may be equally broad, in actuality society usually requires some type of psychotic misunderstanding or an exceptionally crippled lack of control. Not so with the sexual psychopath laws. The general expectation is that most of these individuals will not be psychotic but will have abberrations of character that cause them to act the way they do. Whereas personality disorders will rarely suffice in the insanity defense, they are the rule in sex commitments.

In the second place, the specific mental characteristics necessary for inclusion in the circle of mentally ill sex offenders are usually impairments in the urge functions. Essentially, professionals ask, "Could he or she have controlled himself or herself?" And since the offenders may look to be not sick in all other respects, there is nothing to go on but the very behavior in question. There is no way that either psychiatrists or society can possibly distinguish between most "sick" sex offenders and the "healthy" ones. There is no basis for either psychiatrists or society's representatives to make the transduction.

Thus, a pseudo-*product* question arises and there is no way of answering it. Therefore, it would seem reasonable to refrain from participating in such evaluations. If the laws were altered, there might be a way to participate without expertise. If specific diagnostic categories of sufficient mental illness were set up, psychiatrists could state whether the offender fits into one of these categories. This is unlikely, however, because the laws are not set up to extend compassion to those whom society feel are sick; they are set up primarily to provide an alternative method of incarcerating those whom society feels are not really so sick.

Sexual psychopath laws have been discussed primarily from the standpoint of the *product* issue. There is much else about them that can be faulted, and the GAP (1977, Chapter 12) recommends that they should be repealed. Sex offenders, like other offenders, should have the right to seek compassion through the usual insanity defense channels.

Mental Illness as a Defense Strategy

Not infrequently, an individual will seek psychiatric treatment, and the psychiatrist discovers that the would-be patient has criminal charges pending. Often, it is the defense attorney who has suggested psychiatric treatment, not because he or she feels the client was in urgent need of treatment, but because the contact with a psychiatrist might strengthen the hand of the defense.

The presenting complaint is usually depression or severe anxiety, often with preoccupation, guilt, and sleep difficulty. Psychiatrists often correctly interpret the motives of the attorney as a sham compassion, and they feel they are being manipulated. This pseudo-*product* situation is not only frequently recognized; it is also sometimes overemphasized. Professionals resent being used and this may cause a reaction of anger. Of course, the best way to strike back at the defendant and his or her attorney is to turn the applicant away. For example some psychiatrists might say, "Come back when your legal problems are settled and I'll help you."

This course of action is not recommended. A person may be both sick and manipulative (Bursten, 1973, Chapter 2). Psychiatrists should be concerned neither with abetting nor thwarting the manipulation. They should not take a moral stand with regard to the strategy of the defense. They should evaluate the individual in the same fashion as they evaluate other applicants for treatment.

However, psychiatrists should make it clear that taking the individual into treatment in no way implies that the offense was a *product of mental illness* for which he or she is being treated or that the individual is too sick to stand trial.

DISCIPLINARY PROCEDURES

Warehousing Undesirables

Szasz (1963, p. 47) states that social disturbance is a crucial issue in determining who will be hospitalized. While this is undoubtedly true, it is not the only reason in the majority of cases. However, there are some instances where it becomes apparent that commitment to or retention in a mental hospital has been used primarily for getting or keeping an undesirable individual out of the community or family in situations where no criminal offense has been committed. The young wanderer described in Chapter One is a case in point. When he was on the road, his family often knew where he was but never made any attempt to tell the authorities to hospitalize him. However, when he came home, although he was not psychotic and he disobeyed no laws, he was an intense embarrassment to his family. They would have him committed.

A classic case in the history of involuntary hospitalization in the United States is that of Mrs. Elizabeth Packard (1875). The wife of a minister, she espoused very different views from those of her husband. Under Illinois law during the 1800s, women could be committed at the request of their husbands without the evidence of insanity ordinarily required if the superintendent of the hospital agreed that she was "insane or distracted." It was Mrs. Packard's contention that her husband had her hospitalized because she was an embarrassment and he wanted to get rid of her. During her hospitalization, Mrs. Packard wrote eloquently (and certainly in a nondistracted fashion) about the circumstances of her admission and detention. Her books were an important factor in prompting a change in the Illinois commitment laws.

Another example of involuntary hospitalization is the case of Mr. Bowden. His hospitalization had been prompted by his delusions that people were after him. At the time, he was hearing persecutory voices. In his panic, he ran to the police for protection, and they committed him to a mental hospital.

After several months of treatment, Mr. Bowden's hallucinations and delusions subsided and he evolved into a somewhat hostile and provocative patient. He no longer wanted his medications, and he began to urge other patients not to take theirs. He became a collector of newspaper clippings and would forage for food in the garbage cans. His bedside was a mess. He seemed to delight in challenging the staff and arguing with them about rules. He befriended a woman patient and caused the hospital no end of worry that they were having sexual relations. He continued this pattern for nine years, during which time his medications were raised, lowered, changed, and often not swallowed by him with no appreciable changes in his behavior. There was never any question of his having further hallucinations or frank delusions, but it was clear from the notes in the chart that the staff felt his odd and often provocative behavior would be as unacceptable on the outside as it was on the inside.

During his stay, the patient had made several attempts to contact an attorney or to reach the newspapers by telephone or mail. These efforts were frustrated by the staff and often resulted in his being given more medication or being shifted to more secure wards (where there were more disturbed patients).

Ultimately, with the aid of a lawyer, Mr. Bowden did secure his freedom. He sued the hospital for violating his civil rights by forcing him to take medications, locking him up, refusing him access to an attorney and visitors, refusing him access to the newspapers, and a variety of other actions. By this time, he was living in a small house in the community (he had a small, independent income). He was taking no medication, and his condition was unchanged. He still collected papers, books, and other articles that others would consider trash. He was quite a sight around town; he was disheveled and always carried a sack with his paper valuables. He became single mindedly interested in the rights of mental patients and would argue about them with anyone on the street who stopped to listen to him. However, he fed himself and took care of his basic needs adequately.

During the proceedings of his lawsuit, one of the defendant

doctors acknowledged that at a previous hospital in an urban setting in another state he had discharged patients like Mr. Bowden. Despite this fact and the fact that some of Mr. Bowden's charges were well substantiated in his hospital record, the jury, drawn from the rural community around the hospital, decided in favor of the defendant hospital and doctors. As the courtroom was emptying, one of the jurors approached a defendant psychiatrist and said, "Keep up the good work with these guys, Doc."

In the ensuing months, on several occasions, when Mr. Bowden would stand in front of the public library and try to strike up a conversation about mental patients' rights, the police would be called, and they would take him to the local mental health center. The center, however, refused to recommit him or to treat him; they would just send him home.

It is uncertain how often hospitalization for the convenience of the community occurs, but it has occurred. Two factors have made it less common than it was about a decade ago. Increasing legal scrutiny and tighter commitment laws have had their effect. In addition, tighter budgets have caused departments of mental health to try to discharge as many people as possible to the community. But it still may occur, and if it does, commitment and retention become pseudo-*product* issues because the hospital is acting as a mirror of the community's outrage rather than its compassion.

The role of the psychiatrist is obvious. Every patient should be evaluated with respect to the same commitment standards as every other patient regardless of community desires or political pressures. Of course, the ultimate transduction in the commitment hearing is made by the judge and he or she does reflect community views. However, judges would have a more difficult time warehousing if all the reports of the psychiatrists were against it. And psychiatrists generally have the power to discharge if they feel that the patient does not meet the commitment standards.

Hangmen

In the discussion of hospitalization of political dissenters, Bukovsky and Gluzman's (1974) classification of psychiatrists into Phillistines, Hangmen, and other types was mentioned. The

Hangmen are those who know that they are imprisoning people in mental hospitals, not because they are sick but because the State wants them held there. This, by definition, is a pseudo-*product* situation because the psychiatrist is well aware that the evaluation of the patient is prompted only by sham compassion. The line between warehousing undesirables and Hangmen is thin. If there is a difference at all it is that the Hangman's victims are not generally undesirable in habits or appearance; if it were not for their political views, they would be tolerated in the community.

Perhaps the more important distinction is between the Hangman and the Phillistine. A psychiatrist who has been taught a psychiatric party line that fits in with the prevailing political ideology is not sufficiently independent of thought to question it. All psychiatrists are Phillistines to some extent because they tend to support the prevailing societal ideology. The Phillistine, however, is confronted with a genuine *product* question; using society's standards of illness, he or she participates in a commitment proceeding as described in Chapter Seven.

There are Hangmen in all countries, some with national impact and others on more restricted regional scenes. The case in the United States of Ezra Pound, described by Szasz (1963, Chapter 16) sounds very much like Hangmen, a view shared by Robitscher (1980, pp. 106ff.) and many others. Pound was an American poet and essayist who was in Italy during World War II. While there, he broadcast propaganda for the Axis powers. On his return to America following the war, he was charged with treason, but he was found incompetent to stand trial and was committed to a mental hospital where he stayed for thirteen years, despite the fact that there was no treatment for him and he was not considered dangerous. His eccentricities and idiosyncrasies had been well known for many years before his hearing, but the issue came to a head only in the context of the treason issue. At the hearing, which technically dealt with his competence to stand trial, both government and defense attorneys made apparent their desire that he be found incompetent. Even the judge, in his charge to the jury, made it plain that he favored commitment. The interested reader would find Szasz's description quite revealing. Needless to say, it is not recommended that psychiatrists participate in Hangmen situations.

Disciplining Criminal Offenders

The disciplinary situation to be described here has much in common with warehousing and Hangmen; here, however, an offense has been committed and the trial has been held. The people in this category are those found not guilty by reason of insanity. After the trial, the individual is sent to a mental hospital for observation and evaluation usually for not less than sixty days. If he or she is found presently to meet the criteria for commitment, the hospitalization continues until such time that the commitment criteria are no longer met (*Bolton u Harris*, 1968). In some states, when the hospital declares the patient ready for release, the criminal court judge may hold a hearing and decide that the patient is not yet ready. There are three points about these post-trial procedures which suggest that they may be a pseudo-*product* situation. First, the sixty-plus day evaluation period is unduly long. In this day and age, most acute care mental hospitals keep their new patients about two or three weeks. This period includes both diagnosis and treatment. Unless one is awaiting crucial records from another institution, the evaluation of those found guilty by reason of insanity should be complete in a few days to a week, and those not meeting the commitment standards should be discharged. The remainder of the time is merely disciplinary.

In the second place, the review by the judge before discharge represents society's outrage toward the offenders and toward hospitals that are releasing them "too soon." A peculiar situation can be created in which the doctors say there is no need for further hospitalization while the judge mandates continued hospitalization. What are the psychiatrists to treat? Clearly, the judge is reflecting society's fear of dangerousness. If the individual is dangerous, but the psychiatrists believe he or she no longer meets the mental illness standard (really the incompetence standard as described in Chapter Seven), why does the judge not incarcerate the person in a jail? Because the individual has been not found guilty of a crime, the only legal place of incarceration is in a mental hospital. There have been proposals to extend this judicial review of discharges to ordinary, civilly committed patients as well. There is a real danger that mental hospitals could become quasi prisons—

institutions for the preventive detention of those who have once met the commitment criteria of mental illness but now are detained only because society's representatives are frightened of them.

The third situation that points to the pseudo-*product* nature of some posttrial hospitalizations occurs when an individual with a personality disorder is found not guilty by reason of insanity. This does not occur very often, but it does happen. Occasionally, people with narcissistic, borderline, or schizoid personalities are found commitable after a successful insanity plea. However, many hospitals receiving such patients would not recommend commitment for people with similar personality types who were threatening harm but had not actually done anything. Often the attitude toward this person is, "Do it and you can't cop out by saying you're crazy; you're not crazy enough to be admitted here." The commitment standards, elastic as they are, are sometimes stretched in the face of possible public outrage when a jury has found an individual not guilty by reason of insanity.

In order to understand the pseudo-*product* nature of some of these hospitalizations, the distinction between the adjudication of an insanity plea in a criminal trial and the evaluation of eligibility for commitment must be kept in mind. The obvious distinction is that the insanity plea speaks to the individual's mental state at the time of the offense, while the commitment hearing deals with the individual at present. More importantly, for the point of view of this book, however, is the fact that society's representatives, the jury, have compassion with regard to the offensive behavior when it acquits by reason of insanity. In the commitment hearings that follow, there is still a strong residue of outrage (with its fear component), and the compassion shown by hospitalizing the patient may be a sham.

As in the case of warehousing and Hangmen, psychiatrists should not endorse pseudo-*product* hospitalizations. Each prospective patient should be evaluated within the same circle of criteria as other patients and the psychiatrist's report should not be influenced by social and political pressures. This is easier said than done because the hospitals and psychiatrists most likely to be involved are paid by the state and are part of a mental health system, the director of which is politically appointed. Direct or indirect political pressure often comes with the job.

The observer may look for certain clues in attempting to discern whether a particular hospitalization is a warehouse, Hangmen, or criminal punishment. One should be alerted to this possibility if the individual is being treated exceptionally. By looking at other hospitalized patients, the observer can form a rough idea of the circle that defines mentally ill people who require hospitalization. If the person's diagnosis does not fit within that circle, he or she may have been hospitalized for disciplinary purposes. Further, even if the diagnosis does fall within the circle, if the patient is hospitalized for an unusually long time or with unusual security (usually called restriction of privileges) for people with that particular diagnosis, this may be a disciplinary hospitalization. These conditions are merely alerting points, however, because certain psychiatric situations may justify exceptional treatment.

Several states have been concerned that many patients who have been committed either directly or after a successful insanity plea are treated, discharged, go off their medications, and repeat the kinds of behavior that caused society alarm in the first place. Oregon (O. R. S. Sec. 161.295–161.346) places those found not guilty by reason of insanity under the supervision of a Psychiatric Security Board for a time equal to the maximum sentence for the crime involved. If the individual does not need hospitalization, he or she still may be subject to mandatory outpatient treatment under the Board's ultimate supervision. Other states are also fashioning mandatory outpatient treatment laws, not only for those who have been acquitted by reason of insanity but also for those who are repeatedly civilly hospitalized. The theory is that these people have mental illness in remission and are likely to become dangerous because of mental illness if they go off their medication. This, too, is a pseudo-*product* situation aimed primarily at preventing dangerous behavior rather than at caring for the sick—outrage rather than compassion. Most of the people pressured into treatment under provisions such as these are indeed in remission; they have regained their competence to make decisions. If they were in the hospital, it is doubtful that they could legally be forced to take medications against their will. In these situations, however, the psychiatrist is within professional expertise in predicting that if the individual goes off the medication, he or she is likely to decompensate and act similarly to the way he or she did in the past. Even though the activity is disciplinary, it is also medical. The psychiatrist, of course, should not state that the patient is incompetent to make his or her own decisions. The basic problem with this pseudo-*product* situation does not lie with the evaluations of the psychiatrist; rather it is a matter for legal scrutiny.

At the time of this writing, the Supreme Court has handed down a decision that further legalizes the disciplinary use of psychiatry (*Jones u United States,* 1983). In essence, the Court has stated that if a person has been found not guilty by reason of insanity, he or she may be indefinitely kept in a mental hospital. Commitment hearings must be held periodically, but the guidelines of these hearings make it easier to commit these people than those who have not committed a crime. The Court felt justified in making it easier to detain these people, not because of a present finding of mental illness, but because a person "whose mental illness was sufficient to commit a crime is likely to remain ill and in need of treatment." This mixture of past crimes and present commitability probably represents the societal swing toward outrage described in Chapter Six. The Court also approved the lengthy evaluation period described previously. Additionally, this ruling is the precedent for using exceptional coercive measures on those who are "likely to need treatment." This is the reasoning used in the enforced outpatient treatment situations.

Keeping A Quiet Ward

Chapter Seven briefly discussed the fact that in mental hospitals medications are sometimes used not as a vehicle of compassion for disturbed patients who are incompetent to make their own decisions, but as a vehicle for ward order and discipline. This does not refer to the administration of medicine on a regular basis at a dose level calculated to relieve the psychosis. It does refer to the medication that is administered on a one-time basis when the patient shows disturbed (or disturbing) behavior.

There are two interrelated factors involved in these situations.

The first is the conditions on the ward that may induce agitated behavior on the part of patients. Sometimes such behavior is provoked by other patients and by staff; it may be difficult to evaluate whether a patient's irritation should be allocated to his or her mental illness or to a reasonable reaction to provocation. Beyond that, the ward atmosphere and the number and quality of nursing staff play a part in determining the number and intensity of disturbed behaviors on the unit. Chapter Seven referred to the economic considerations that underlie the shameful understaffing in many public, mental hospitals.

The second factor has to do with the way these disturbances are handled. Not infrequently, psychiatrists will leave an order in the patient's chart indicating that the nurse (often not even a registered nurse) may give a dose of psychotropic medication "p. r. n. agitation," as the need arises for agitated behavior (Bursten, 1980; *Davis u Hubbard,* 1980). The decision to medicate is not made on the basis of the psychiatrist's evaluation that the behavior in question is a *product of mental illness* but often on the nurse's desire to quell the disturbance. Doctors like quiet wards because this cuts down on the frequency with which they are called to the unit; nurses like quiet wards even more because they live there eight hours a day, and there is always the danger that an outburst will be contagious among patients or will lead to violence. Often, then, the medication is administered as a disciplinary measure without much consideration about whether the agitation is a *product of mental illness.*

To some extent, this process is inevitable, because even the most searching attempts to allocate the behavior between sick and healthy aspects of the patient will not yield a clear-cut answer. However, with more appropriate budgets, hospitals could provide enough of the right kind of personnel to listen to the patient who is agitated and to attempt to settle a provocative social situation without the use of what must be called tranquilization. Further, if the agitated patient were seen as posing a genuine *product* question, the decision would be made by the psychiatrist rather than delegated to sometimes minimally trained staff. In this situation, while the treatment of agitated patients should be a genuine *product* situation, it is sometimes handled as a pseudo-*product* situation—a disciplinary practice.

Psychiatric Dismissals From Employment

In Chapter One, Mr. Donovan's case, the argumentative man who irritated his supervisors in a federal agency by accusing them of using government property for their individual gains, was described. Since his work performance was excellent, the agency was loathe to fire him. In addition, the supervisors correctly surmised that he might be the type to sue. They were hoping he would be declared medically unfit to work. This was a pseudo-*product* request. They did not have compassion for the employee; they wanted a psychiatrist to be a hatchet man.

Essentially, the psychiatrist gave a descriptive evaluation. However, no statement was made relative to Mr. Donovan's fitness to work. The position taken in these cases, even if the patient is psychotic, is that it is up to the officials at the company to make the transduction. Only they can decide if such people are too sick to work. (The reader should keep in mind that even people with psychosis are employable.)

In this manner, the pseudo-*product* request is sidestepped and it is turned back to them as a genuine *product* issue about which they must make the transduction.

The General Hospital Disciplinarian

Not infrequently, doctors on other medical specialty services of a general hospital will turn to the psychiatrist for help when their patients misbehave. Their motivation, like the motivation of the ward staff in some mental hospitals, is to have a quiet unit with compliant patients. Despite the fact that the evaluation request is not made compassionately, the psychiatrist should evaluate the situation and make whatever suggestions are helpful. Often with older patients, the disturbing behavior will diminish if the psychiatric medications used to "calm" the patient are reduced. Other patients may have things on their minds that they need to talk about. Or the psychiatrist may see social situations on the ward that are provocative. Some patients may be acutely psychotic and need psychotropic drugs. Others may be having psychiatric manifestations of the medicines that are being used to treat the illness which brought them to the hospital or of the illness, itself. Still others may need good firm limit setting.

The situation here is similar to that of the manipulative patient who is sent over by his or her attorney as part of the defense strategy. Even though it is a pseudo-*product* situation, the patient and the situation should be evaluated in the same manner as any other patient. If treatment is indicated, it should be offered.

THIRD PARTY COVERAGE

The types of conditions seen by the consumer as sick and the cost of treatments for these conditions tend to expand to the degree that others (third parties) pay for the service (Enthoven, 1980, pp. 9ff.). Since the resources of these payers are not unlimited, some method of determining who gets what must be devised. In part, this determination is accomplished by defining which conditions count as payable ones.

Third party payers may be public or private. The public ones are state or national governments; there may be blanket health plans for all citizens or more limited ones, such as the social security disability programs discussed in Chapter Eight. Private plans include a variety of health insurance plans in which a premium is paid to the insurance company that pays all the covered bills, employee assistance plans in which industry buys certain health services, and alternative financing and delivery systems, such as prepaid group plans, in which the doctors agree to provide for the comprehensive health needs of subscribers at a monthly fee (Enthoven, 1980, Chapter 4).

In Chapter Eight, the process of *deciding the individual case* in social security adjudications was discussed. The circle of allowable mental illnesses is often so vaguely defined that disputes about whether a person is sick (or sick enough to qualify) may arise. This is decided by an administrative hearing or an appeals court and the tension between compassion and indifference weigh heavily in the decision. These are genuine *product* issues and they are similar in the private sector.

What is of interest here are the *standards*, or more generally the *guidelines* for describing the circle of covered illnesses and payments.

More particularly, interest will be focused not on which specific mental illnesses are covered, but on the degree to which mental illnesses in general are covered.

As Tancredi and Slaby (1977, pp. 126ff.) point out, compared to other major health problems, such as cancer, mental health research and treatment receives a disproportionately small amount of support from the federal government. Private third party payers stringently limit their expenditures for psychiatric care by paying a lesser percentage of each bill by limiting the amount of treatment for which the patient will receive benefits, and sometimes by excluding psychiatric coverage altogether. Where states have mandated that private insurers cover mental illness, the reimbursement to psychiatrists is often proportionately lower than to other medical specialists. The insistence that private payers cover mental illness is not necessarily a compassionate bow to the needs of the sick; it may be a means of helping the state get out of the mental health business altogether (Stoddard et al., 1983).

What are the *competing interests* lying behind this tendency to limit mental health coverage? On the one hand, of course, there is always a tendency for payers to want to reduce costs. This is a reflection of indifference—let people take care of themselves. It is when the other side is examined—that which impels any payout for mental illness—that the question arises of whether the degree to which mental illness is covered reflects a genuine or pseudo-*product* decision.

All plans must distribute their finite resources among the various illnesses according to certain principles (called *distributive justice*). If the available funds were distributed among the various kinds of illness according to the principle of need (Galston, 1980, Chapter 6), it would imply that compassion underlies the distribution principle. In this situation, mental illness would probably fare better than it does. Tancredi and Slaby suggest that the funds are allocated on the principle of what Galston describes as a desert— nonmentally ill people seem to deserve a greater share of the funds because they more often give promise of returning to productive lives in society. If this were so, the decision to include mental illness as a sufficiently important illness to fund (falling within the circle of fundable illnesses) would be a pseudo-*product* decision because it would not depend on compassion but on the cold economic calculations. Indeed, the response of psychiatry to the underfunding is often an economic one; professionals attempt to show that the costs are not so high and the economic benefits may be substantial.

While such factors may indeed operate, the most important principle underlying the distribution of health resources is the principle of market value (Posner, 1981, pp. 60.ff.). The provider will cover what the purchaser will pay for. Once again, the decision is an economic one, and, from the provider's point of view, compassion does not enter into the decision.

However, there is an undercurrent of the tension between true compassion and indifference in the allocation decision. If the major distribution principle is market value (with desert playing a secondary role), people must be asked why they not willing to bargain harder (pay proportionately more) for psychiatric care. Or, to put it in simpler terms, why do the consumers not demand better psychiatric coverage, even if coverage of some other illnesses may need to be reduced? The answer lies in the strangeness the public feels about psychiatric illness. There is relatively little compassion toward psychiatric sickness when compared with other illnesses. If this were not so the public would not tolerate the disgraceful conditions of its mental hospitals. In part, compassion implies putting oneself in the other person's shoes; it is not as easily aroused toward mental illness as it is toward cancer or birth defects.

To grasp the effect of compassion on market value, one need only examine the role the media played in stirring compassion for those needing liver transplants. The cost per case of this treatment is very high; it is a very expensive procedure in terms of allocation of resources but one where demand was roused by a compassion that spread to the halls of Congress and to the President, himself.

Although the issue is by no means clear, whether mental illness will fall within the circle of sufficiently ill to merit funding only appears to be a pseudo-*product* issue, and to attempt to discuss it chiefly in terms of economic impact may miss the point. The role of compassion in determining the market value of sickness is sufficient to conclude that the decision to include or exclude psychiatric illness as significantly fundable may be a genuine *product* issue after all. And psychiatrists may need to pay increasing attention to emotional appeals—to arousing compassion—if the market-value of the product is to increase.

CHAPTER ELEVEN

COMPASSION—COMPASSION
The Scope of Psychiatry

All the *product* situations described in the preceding chapters require psychiatrists to decide whether the behavior in question is to be called sick or whether another label of deviance would be more appropriate. In Chapters Two and Three, it was pointed out how the definitions of sickness fail to give the guidance needed to make these decisions, especially in the many borderline situations confronted in society. In Chapter Four, the view was put forth that these decisions may be guided primarily by emotions, and this book has attempted to show that compassion prompts a judgement of sickness while outrage and indifference prompt judgements of other kinds of deviance.

However, there are behaviors that, while eliciting compassion, generally are not considered to be *products of illness*. In the preceding chapter, the situation was encountered where the prosecutor has compassion for the "nice" middle-class shoplifter; the district attorney feels that he or she was unwise, not sick. Likewise, although the actions of children are felt to be unwise or inexperienced, the compassion felt for them does not lead to a judgement of illness. The plight of the poor and downtrodden may stir compassion but their activities are not characterized as products of illness. Instead, they may not be given a deviant label, or they may be characterized as unfortunate. Their actions may be thought praiseworthy under the circumstances. The clergy treat sinners or those who transgress with compassion; they want to help them, but they do not feel they are sick.

In Chapter Four the ways deviant people are classified were discussed; society holds all types of deviant individuals responsible for the behavior in question with the exception of the sick and the inexperienced. The two categories were separated by the notion that the helplessness of the sick comes from within because of a crippled choosing mechanism, while the inexperienced have intact choosing mechanisms but a deficiency of inputs from outside. However, the helplessness of both states elicits compassion; on what basis is it determined that one class has a crippled choosing mechanism while the other does not?

Apparently, while compassion may be a necessary ingredient for a judgement of illness, it is not sufficient. There will be many situations where psychiatrists have compassion for people, where it is felt that they need whatever help can be given, and where professionals will still have to struggle with a *sick or sinful? sick or inexperienced?*, or *sick or unwise* (in the sense of needing guidance)?, or even *sick or deprived?* question. When the alternative to treating the person as sick is not to punish or to leave him or her alone but to provide significant help, the situation is conceptualized as the tension between compassion and compassion; essentially the decision hinges on the tension between compassion in two different contexts.

This is not merely an academic problem. The subject matter of psychiatry generally is considered to be mental illness. While psychiatry is one of the helping professions, there are many other helping professions, such as social work, law, financial advising, the clergy, etc. All of them are concerned with thoughts, feelings, and especially behaviors of people. But psychiatry differs from the others because its province is sick thoughts, feelings, and behaviors. Psychiatrists have patients; other helping professionals have clients, parishioners, or students. Therefore, the very definition of psychiatry, itself — its scope, what its consumers can expect and to some degree what its sponsors will pay for, which activities will be considered to be legitimate — seems to be linked to *sick or _____?* questions.

ILLNESS REVISITED

Many writers discuss the scope of psychiatry — and, indeed, the scope of medicine — as if the crucial concepts were obvious and their meanings enjoyed universal agreement. Doctors, including psychiatrists, deal with disease and everyone knows what that is.

However, already seen in Chapter Two, the nature and concept of disease is both complicated and slippery. Part of the difficulty lies in certain philosophical, and especially logical, features of the way the term, *disease* is used (Fabrega, 1972).

One such problem arises because some people view disease as an entity, an actual thing that exists in nature, as it were. Others view it as an abstraction, as a human way of classifying clusters of things and events; while these things and events may occur in nature, disease is the way people classify them.

On the one hand, writers such as Cassell (1976, p. 48) state that disease means "a disturbance of the organs or body fluids characterized by structural alteration or biochemical change." In a similar vein, Levine (1978) defines disease as an entity that is characterized by abnormalities of bodily structure or function.

On the other hand, Riese (1953, p. 62 and p. 88), while granting the reality of the data of organ structures and functions, says that disease is a product of the way professionals think about and organize these data. Engel (1960) echoes this view.

I agree with the latter group of writers. There is a wide variety of human structures and functions in the real world; doctors mentally collect certain types of them and call them disease. Disease, then, is not a state existing in reality; it refers to a way of classifying data derived from reality. A circle can be drawn around certain things that are observed and the disease label is applied to the area bounded by the circle. Whether such a structure or such a function or even such a behavior is disease is a matter of policy rather than a matter of fact. And, indeed, as the definitions of those who hold that diseases are entities are scrutinized more closely, a flaw can be detected in their reasoning. For even they do not state that diseases are structures or functions; for them diseases are *abnormalities* or *alterations* or *disturbances* of structures and functions. In other words, they are *types* of realities — classes. This type of classification will be reconsidered to shortly.

Another problem that makes the understanding of disease so slippery is the failure to distinguish disease as a concept or general class from specific diseases which carry specific diagnostic labels. Within the circle of things and events that are called disease are various subgroups, such as tuberculosis, peptic ulcer, hypertension, mania, etc. These are the specific diseases, and as Feinstein

(1968) has pointed out, they too are classifications rather than entities. While each of these specific diseases has its own defining characteristics, what ties them all together within the circle of things called disease is a set of common characteristics that define disease as a concept.

Hence the relationship between disease and illness is brought into focus. Those writers, such as Cassell (1976, Chapter 2) and Levine (1978) who maintain that disease is an entity, attempt to distinguish between illness and disease. Illness refers to the person and how that person feels; he or she is ill. Disease refers to the abnormal organs; the person *has* disease. Since I maintained that the word disease refers to a way of classifying clusters of characteristics rather than to an entity, the way a person feels is one of the characteristics of the disease in question. One may say that a person is ill or diseased. One may also say that a person has an illness or a disease, so long as one is aware that the terms describe classes, not things. In addition, Cassell and Levine are confusing specific diseases with the general class of diseases. It is true that often organs are observed to determine which specific disease is present. But the organ is called diseased only if it has specific effects on the person.

One thing that often underlies the disagreement about whether illness and disease should be separated or united is a difference in the way the mind-body relationship is viewed. In Chapter Two, both the interactionist and identity viewpoints and their implications for the definition of disease were described. Most of the writers who argue that disease is an entity and is exclusive of the way the person feels seem to draw a sharp line between the biological and the psychological. In this view, diseases are abnormalities of the body that may interact with but are of a different nature from the mind. My preference is for the identity viewpoint that maintains that a change in the mind is a change in the body — psychological is biological. In this book, as stated in Chapter One, the terms illness and disease are used interchangeably.

Now, all specific illnesses have a set of common characteristics that define the general class or concept of illness. This set of common characteristics must be distinguished from explanations of disease. Riese (1953) has described a variety of explanations of disease that have been in use through the ages. These include possession by evil spirits, punishment for moral transgression, disturbance of the balance of humors or elements of nature or the vital forces, and disturbance of structures and functions. All these explanations assume that the common characteristics of disease are known. The circle has been defined, and now it must be explained what happened to place an individual (or an organ system) within it.

What are these common characteristics that define the boundaries of the circle of diseases? If they are matters of policy, they can be whatever people want them to be so long as they are useful and they communicate something to others (Bursten, 1982b). Some of them have been discussed in Chapter Two: undesirability, a natural process, a biological process, a greater individual than social focus, and inability to change the characteristics by willpower. In Chapter Four, a basic characteristic of the compassion-eliciting effect of the characteristics on others was added. But since all of these characteristics could also apply to the behavior of children "who don't know any better," some additional characteristics are needed, which will keep common specific diseases within the circle while excluding such conditions as childish behavior.

One approach might be to use adjectives such as those employed by Cassell, Levine, and by most interaction theorists. Diseases are characterized by abnormal, altered, disturbed, or even dysfunctional structures and processes; childish behavior is normal, even if bothersome. But what constitutes abnormality? Why is a diastolic blood pressure of 100 disturbed while a pressure of 85 is not? Why is a liver with tumor cells abnormal while a liver without such cells is not? One current theory suggests that depression is caused by a lowered activity of certain chemical messengers in the brain. Why is that level of activity a disturbance while the somewhat higher level is not?

People apply these adjectives and the label of disease to those conditions that threaten them in certain ways. The capacity to elicit anxiety is the additional characteristic needed to separate the compassion-eliciting disease from the compassion-eliciting nonill behavior of children.

If the condition is not frightening—or is not potentially frightening, it is not an illness. A person (or an organ, for that matter) is classified as diseased only if the structure or function under study can lead to frightening consequences if unattended to. This is the characteristic that distinguishes between a diastolic pressure of 100 and one of 85, between a liver with tumor cells and one with a whole variety of cells but no cancerous ones, between depression and lowered chemical functioning and the absence of depression and somewhat higher chemical functioning. If there were no frightening consequences, a diastolic pressure of 100 would not be considered abnormal, etc. Like a seven-foot tall man, it might be considered unusual, but not pathological.

Cassell (1976, Chapter 2) has given some clues about the nature of this anxiety. Part of feeling sick (he would say "ill") is the threat to the sense of bodily integrity and intactness (the sense of self), the sense of being somewhat disconnected from the group (or sometimes, the world), the failure of the sense of indestructibility, and the loss of the sense of being able to control these events. The loss of the sense of control is particularly noteworthy because it leads to the fact that people labelled as sick are not held responsible for their signs and symptoms. These threats are powerful and they are related to an understanding of who and where persons are in the scheme of things. The anxiety attendant to this situation is close to what the existentialists (Binswanger, 1949) refer to as existential anxiety, and that term will be used to differentiate it from the many more specific anxieties concerning particular social situations. Like compassion, existential anxiety is part of the sociobiological heritage. In fact, it is because of this basic anxiety that humans can be compassionate — suffering with — along with those who are experiencing it more strongly. Compassion in the context of existenial anxiety impels a condition to be classified as an illness.

Mental illness is somewhat set apart from other illnesses. In the case of peptic ulcers, existential anxiety is stirred by the disruptions of the relationship to the scheme of things. For example, bodily integrity and the sense of control of destiny are challenged. However, with mental illness, the very functions with which people place themselves in the order of things lose their bearings. They may lose control over their ability to control anything, so to speak. If they are disoriented, they seem to fear that they have lost their ability to know even if they were once again to be related to the universe. With the ulcers, an intact mind can know its disrupted relationships. With mental illness, the organ of knowing, itself, may be hampered.

Is it any wonder that in more primitive times medicine and religion were one and the same (Sigerist, 1941, Chapter 1)? Existential anxiety is important in both disciplines. Both Riese and Engle have noted how tenaciously the entity concept of disease appears time and again through history. It seems quite possible that the idea of an entity "in there" that is a disease is a reflection of the evil spirits which possessed the "less rational" ancients and threatened to destroy their comfortable relation with the universe. It is remarkable that they ever managed to separate. And there is still overlap. Most scientists view acquired immune deficiency syndrome as a disease whose natural causes are potentially understandable; however, many biblical literalists view it as God's way of punishing homosexual men. And hospitals still remain as one of the largest enterprises of various religious groups; the marriage of hospitals and churches seems quite reasonable (really, quite emotional).

To recapitulate: disease is not a thing; it is a class of conditions sharing common characteristics. As such, it is not a matter of fact but a matter of policy. People decide which conditions shall be included in the class and which conditions shall be excluded. The criteria by which that decision is made includes those listed in Chapter Two. More basic, however, is the capacity of the included conditions to elicit compassion in the context of existential anxiety.

THE GRADIENT OF MENTAL ILLNESS

As discussed in Chapter Two, some clusters of mental characteristics unequivocally seem to qualify as illness; however, many others are quite equivocal. Some writers, such as Torrey (1974), have attempted to distinguish between disease and problems of living. Torrey presented twenty-eight clusters of mental characteristics that are likely to come to the attention of the psychiatrist, and essentially he divided them into those with demonstrated or presumed brain disease (illness) and the others (problems in living). He then concluded that since brain disease was the province of neurologists and neurosurgeons and problems of living were not sickness altogether, there is nothing left for psychiatrists to do but to pack their bags and leave the scene.

In making this distinction, Torrey relied on an interactionist approach that distinguishes between psychological and biological processes. My disagreement with that approach was discussed in the previous section. However, his style of presenting the argument is a good one and will be employed here. Many of the disorders listed in DSM III will be presented; these are the clusters of mental characteristics with which the psychiatrist may be confronted. Here, they will be discussed in terms of the criteria of illness.

However, some preliminary remarks are necessary. At the outset, there will be general agreement that these clusters of mental characteristics may meet the criteria listed in Chapter Two and that they can elicit compassion. It seems that where they differ from one another is primarily on the dimension of existential anxiety. Those clusters that stir little existential anxiety may also evoke a low level of compassion, and people may be less inclined' to agree that the other criteria of illness have been met. On the other hand, those conditions eliciting considerable existential anxiety also evoke considerable compassion and are more likely to invoke the concept of illness.

The degree of undesirability, in particular, is probably directly related to the amount of existential anxiety that is stirred. This is what is meant when people talk about illnesses which are serious and those which are not so serious. It is probably not useful to consider undesirable behavior in terms of either illness or nonillness. Instead, it would be better to speak of a gradient of illness. The element that locates any cluster of mental characteristics on this gradient is the degree of existential anxiety it evokes. Those clusters that elicit little existential anxiety are not at all serious illnesses; society may prefer to classify people with these conditions as criminal, unwise, lazy, manipulative, unpleasant, or inexperienced. Sin is a special case and it will be considered in a later section of this chapter. Those people whose conditions elicit a high degree of existential anxiety are quite severely ill, and it is much less likely that they will be put into the other categories. This concept of a gradient of illness holds for other classes of disease as well. Indigestion is very little illness, peptic ulcers are more serious, and a person with cancer of the stomach is considered to be even more severly ill.

Actually, since mental illness is not a thing (which one can have more or less of) but a classification, to be consistent, people should not speak of degrees of illness but rather of degrees of similarity to the definers of the illness category or to the degree of comfort in placing the cluster of characteristics in question in that category. However, it is easier to stay with the more common usage and speak of a gradient of illness. A review of the various conditions in terms of the patient or someone who knows him or her well can demonstrate how the illnesses are arrayed along the gradient.

Rated at the top of the gradient (Grade 5), would be dementias, deliria, and the psychoses. Dementias result from deterioration of the brain cells due to a variety of causes. Deliria are more transient alterations in brain function due to reversible physiological conditions. The orientation and ability to place oneself in surroundings and the ability to think clearly about a situation are diminished in these conditions. The psychoses (schizophrenia, the affective disorders, such as mania and severe depression, and paranoid disorders) also generate considerable existential anxiety. Even if people with these conditions know where they are, they cannot well place themselves in the contexts of their situations, and often their behavior is incongruent with their situations. This is a serious breach in the relationship with the order of things.

Amnesias would be assigned to Grade 4. People with amnesia generally act well related to their situations; their disruptions are with their pasts or histories. A sense of continuity with oneself is essential to one's existential well-being.

Grade 3 (moderate severity) has several types of conditions. The various illnesses wherein the patient is convinced he or she has a nonmental (somatic) disease fall in this category. These include hypochondriasis, psychogenic pain, and conversion disorder (all of which have been described elsewhere in this book). People with these conditions are oriented and have continuity but raise questions about bodily integrity and vulnerability. There is always the possibility that the doctor who did not find anything was wrong. And if he or she were right, there is something unsettling about a sense of self so out of touch with its body.

Various anxiety disorders are also included in Grade 3. People with these conditions, while oriented to their situations, are plagued by alien forces, the anxiety effect of which they can actually feel and which prevent them from relating the way they would like to. This anxiety seems to limit the power and ability to control.

Sexual inhibitions and impulse disorder would be placed in Grade 2. While inhibited sexual function does represent some loss of bodily control and integrity, it seems so much more limited than the illnesses in the higher grades. Most of the body is intact, and, in contrast to the somatizing illnesses of Grade 3, there does not seem to be the disruption of the relationship of self to body. The sex organs actually do not work well, and the self knows it. Impulse disorders (shoplifting, fire setting, etc.) appear to be so intentional to the casual observer that they do not even seem to belong to Grade 2. It is only when one gets to know the individual well that one can sense the build-up of tension that seems to erupt in the activity which suggests a loss of control.

The category of psychological factors affecting physical conditions probably also belongs in Grade 2. Here, there are somatic illness, such as ulcers, asthma, headaches, etc., and they are made worse when the person is stressed. Once again, the disruption of bodily integrity is limited, and although the patient knows what makes it worse (stress), he or she does not seem to be able to control it.

Perhaps chronic alcohol and drug users should be included in Grade 2. If they have not deteriorated (dementia), they seem to be acting out of intentionality, but, like people with impulse disorders, it is also possible to feel that they have a loss of control.

The lowest grade may be numbered 1, although some people would assign it a 0. Here, the adjustment disorders and the personality disorders are characterized.

Although adjustment disorders seem to be merely responses to the stresses and strains of living and should give rise to virtually no existential anxiety, as seen in Chapter Nine, some people have unusually strong reactions and some seem overly vulnerable. These people may indeed sense that their lives are not in their own hands. Given a chance in a good psychotherapeutic situation, people with certain personality disorders will reveal their existential anxiety. For example, some borderline people suffer from fleeting lapses in their sense of self. Schizotypal people may sense wierd, unearthy presences. Even people whose personalities do not include such problems may seek help because of a vague malaise or perhaps a chronic maladjustment that signals to them that their life is not in order or has no meaning. These may be low level existential anxieties compared to those in the other groups, and this is why the question of whether these conditions should be called disease is subject to such argument.

Placing certain clusters of mental characteristics in the middle or lower grades does not imply that they are of lesser importance. The people whose conditions fall in Grade 3, whether or not they should be considered ill, have a very significant impact on the total amount of money expended for medical care. People with Grade 1 conditions may have serious negative impact on their own lives, their families, and others with whom they come into contact. The lower grade refers only to seriousness along the illness gradient. For example, with little existential anxiety, a cluster of characteristics may not be seen as serious illness while it may be seen as serious crime.

Of course, not everyone would agree with the way the various conditions have been arranged along the gradient. What is important is not how they are arrayed but that they can be put in an order. This gradient underlies the concept of sufficient mental illness used throughout this book. However, sufficiency has no meaning in the abstract. As already seen, sufficiency in one context is not necessarily sufficiency in another. Sufficiency gains meaning when the question is asked, "Sufficient to trigger what?" In terms of the issue relevant to this chapter, the answer must be, "Sufficient to trigger the attention of the psychiatrist." If mental illness is the subject matter of psychiatry, do psychiatrists deal with all such illnesses or only with those that are sufficiently serious? Is the scope of the profession more broadly or more narrowly defined? And who is to be the transducer who can take a particular degree of existential anxiety generated by a certain condition and use it to answer the question, "Is this how scared one should feel in order to use a psychiatrist?"

In contrast with many of the situations considered previously, there is no formally constituted group of society's policymakers that could balance competing interests and come out with standards for determining if a cluster of mental characteristics is sufficiently sick to fall within the purview of psychiatry. Psychiatry as an organized profession has a wide divergence of opinion about the matter. The implication of the gradient of mental illness is that even if it is agreed that the subject matter of psychiatry is people with mental illness, there is no logical way to determine the scope of psychiatry on the basis of this subject matter. The scope is decided by the inclinations of individual psychiatrists and the market forces that bring patients with various degrees of illness to them.

MODELS OF HELPGIVING

The scope of psychiatry cannot be defined on the basis that it deals with mental illness. The subject matter of psychiatry poses a *product* dilemma and there are no rules for resolving it. If psychiatry's scope cannot be defined on the basis of its subject· matter, can other criterion be used? One such criterion, which is sometimes suggested, is that of psychiatrists' functions; the scope is defined by what they do. Since psychiatrists are doctors, their scope might be limited to medical functions. In order to pursue this proposition, there must be some understanding of what medical functions are.

The position taken in Chapter Four is that the nature of the emotional reaction to the deviant person in great measure determines whether he or she is held responsible for having produced the cluster of characteristics in question. The decision to assign responsibility to the person for having produced the behavior is part of the intellectual overlay in the way the deviant person is classified. It also plays an important role in determining how psychiatrists will respond to that person. That response will be referred to as helpgiving, although various responses may be more or less helpful.

The response of the helpgiver goes beyond assigning responsibility for having produced the behavior. He or she also assigns obligatory responsibility (Edwards, 1969, pp. 64ff.)—deciding who has the major burden for bringing about the change. In some cases, the helpgiver assumes that responsibility; in other cases he or she acts as a guide but places the major burden of responsibility for producing the change on the deviant person. Several factors determine who shall bear the responsibility for effecting the change. The way the helpseeker presents him or herself evokes a greater or lesser urge on the part of the helpgiver to assume responsibility. The training and ideological adherence of the helpgiver plays a part. The particular personality of the helpgiver inclines him or her to assume a more active or more passive, a more or less authoritarian, a more or less dominant role. Indeed, personality characteristics play a part in determining which profession with which ideology in its training will have been chosen by the helpgiver (Henry et al., 1971).

These two sets of assignment of responsibility—responsibility for having produced the behavior and responsibility for producing the change—are helpful in setting up four models of the helpgiving relationship. Brickman et al. (1982) have gone into some detail about this fourfold construction and this presentation is based on theirs. However, names and attributes of some of the models they presented have been changed in order to adapt their classification for use in this book. These models are types of relationships that are triggered when the helpseeker presents him or herself, or is presented, to the helpgiver.

1. The disciplinary model is triggered when the person in question is considered criminal, unwise (in the sense of carelessness), lazy, manipulative, or unpleasant. These people elicit outrage in varying degrees of intensity. In some cases, the emotional reaction may be sufficiently low to be termed indifference. Their choosing mechanism is assumed to be intact and they are held responsible for having produced the behavior in question. The helpgiver will punish, but then it is the responsibility of the person in question to do better next time. This model is used in some of the situations discussed in Chapter Ten.

2. The educational model is triggered when the person is consid-

ered inexperienced or unwise (in the sense of not knowing how to make better choices). This class has been termed *compensatory* by Brickman et al. in order that it might include people who have been deprived of material as well as informational advantages. The reaction is primarily one of compassion, but it is compassion without existential anxiety. Being inexperienced or unwise does not estrange one from the order of things or make one feel powerless. This is why the choosing mechanism is assumed to be intact. However, these people are not considered to be responsible for having produced the behavior in question; the inexperience resulted most immediately from a lack of input from the environment. While instruction and guidance may be provided, it is the responsibility of the individual to practice and learn.

3. The religious model is triggered when the person is considered to be sinning or transgressing. There is a sequence of emotions here. The initial reaction is outrage, albeit it may be of moderate intensity. This outrage is in the context of existential anxiety; the sinner's relationship to the order of things is disrupted and anchorless because his or her relationship to God is damaged. This complex of emotions probably partly explains why religion and medicine have clung so closely together (existential anxiety) and why they separated (outrage versus compassion). Following the initial emotional reaction, there is compassion as the clergy offer redemption. This sequence is represented by the well-known blame and forgiveness pattern of the clergy. The choosing mechanism is assumed to be intact and the individual is held responsible for having produced the behavior. While it is up to the individual to repent, the ultimate responsibility for changing the person's status lies with the helpgiver—in this case, a member of the clergy who can confer forgiveness.

4. The medical model is triggered by the person who is considered sick. The emotion elicited is compassion in the context of existential anxiety. The person's choosing mechanism is assumed to be crippled and therefore he or she is not held responsible for having produced the behavior in question. While the individual is expected to follow the doctor's advice, the burden of responsibility for the treatment falls most heavily on the physician's shoulders.

It should not be surprising to find that these four models of helpgiving relationships are not entirely separate from each other. The definers of the categories are the assignment of the two types of responsibility. This assignment is part of the intellectual overlay stemming from emotional reactions, and it is rare that emotions occur in pure and unmixed forms.

The models and some of their attributes are presented in tabular form. The attributes listed under each model are by no means exhaustive. The medical model, in particular, has been discussed in considerable detail by Siegler and Osmond (1974). However, in terms of the issues considered in this book, this presentation should suffice.

Table I.

		Helpseeker Responsible for Producing Change	Helpgiver Responsible for Producing Change
		Disciplinary Model	*Religious Model*
	1. Deviancy	Criminal, manipulative, unpleasant, lazy	Sinful
Helpseeker responsible for cluster of characteristics	2. Emotions elicited	Outrage	Blame in context of existential anxiety
	3. Choosing mechanism	Intact	Intact
	4. Helping activity	Punishment	Forgiveness, love, Acceptance
		Educational Model	*Medical Model*
	1. Deviancy	Inexperienced, unwise	Sick
Helpseeker not responsible for cluster of characteristics	2. Emotion elicited	Compassion	Compassion in context of existential anxiety
	3. Choosing mechanism	Intact	Crippled
	4. Helping activity	Education	Treatment

One might argue that the models clearly define the functions. The deviant who is called sick is treated by the medical model and therefore by the doctor. But, there is disagreement about who is called sick. Beyond that consideration, however, even if a person is considered sick, the medical model is not the only one applicable. Consider the man who comes to the doctor because of restlessness, irritability, occasional lightheadedness with ringing in the ears, palpitating heart, and sleep difficulty. A careful history reveals that he drinks several cups of coffee in the morning, sips cola drinks all afternoon, and has tea at night. In the best medical tradition, the doctor makes the diagnosis of caffeinism. This is an illness of Grade 2 to 3 severity. Even the interactionists can be satisfied because the characteristics can be explained by physiological processes. However, the doctor now shifts to the educational model. The treatment of this illness is to teach the patient to stay away from certain offending liquids — to change his dietary habits. Doctors have been engaging in this sort of education for centuries. Indeed, as Adler (1981) has pointed out, medical tasks are only part of what psychiatrists (and other good doctors) have been doing all along. Doctors participate in rehabilitation (which often is an educational task), in social and legal functions, such as those described throughout this book, and even in educational tasks designed to help patients achieve optimal (normal) growth.

Since the treatment of caffeinism uses the educational model, perhaps psychiatrists should say that the person was not sick; he was merely inexperienced. Nevertheless, few would argue that this man was correct in coming to the doctor. Does the scope of psychiatry, then, extend beyond sickness to conditions of inexperience? It seems that the better course is to say that this person was both sick and inexperienced; the existential anxiety (sick) steered him to the psychiatrist and the correction of his inexperience effected the desired change.

In the caffeinism example, education does not act directly on the characteristics in question; instead, the effect on the illness is an indirect one acting through the change in what the patient drinks. However, education, defined broadly as in the case of the educational model, sometimes has the peculiar property of being able to act directly on characteristics considered ill. Biofeedback is a process whereby the individual is able to observe his or her physiological functioning (e.g. blood flow in the fingers) on an electronic monitor. With practice, the patient may learn how to gain a certain amount of control over that physiological function and thus alleviate certain illnesses such as headaches. Other behavioral techniques, such as relaxation training, may also have direct effects. Yet, these procedures fall in the educational rather than the medical model. While the patient is not assigned responsibility for having produced the characteristics in question, he or she is given the burden of producing the change under the guidance of the doctor.

Other illnesses of Grades 1 to 3 severity may be directly treated by educational methods. Some of these methods are behavioral (e.g. not giving social reinforcement to complaints of chronic pain—which sometimes reduces the pain, itself) while some are more conventionally psychotherapeutic. While psychoanalytic therapies are arguably medical or educational, other types of psychotherapy are structured clearly in the educational model (Karasu, 1977; Brickman et al., 1982). Some distressing mental characteristics that seemed so automatic and out of the person's control at the outset are alleviated as the individual gains a sense of mastery over them. Thus, some conditions definable as illness can appropriately trigger the educational model rather than the medical model. Indeed, one can cite examples of some illnesses having triggered the disciplinary and religious models that resulted in a satisfactory outcome. It would seem that nature has little respect for neat classifications. This comes as no surprise to those who maintain that social and psychological processes are, indeed, biological.

PSYCHIATRY'S UNIQUE FUNCTION

If the scope of psychiatry is to be defined by its functions, these functions may be limited arbitrarily to medical ones. Indeed, there are many (Siegler and Osmond, 1974; Schwartz, 1974: Ludwig and Othmer, 1977; Hackett, 1977) who urge that psychiatry return to the medical model. Once again, there is no underlying science that dictates this course; it is a matter of policy decision. From the point of view of functions, the argument states that all the educative functions can be performed by other professionals and psychiatrists should refer people who need these skills to them. The nonmedical functions that psychiatrists perform are not unique. Psychiatrists should stick to the single function which is unique to them — the medical function.

Much of the medical model argument is rhetoric (Bursten, 1979a); furthermore, such a policy would not be salutary for patients or for the profession. If functioning is restricted to the medical model, psychiatrists are likely to misapply medical functions when other functions might be more beneficial. One has only to look at how physicians dole out antianxiety medications by the bushelful to people who are described by some psychiatrists as having "problems in living." One tends to do what one has been trained to do; "trained only medical" may mean "treat only medical."

Nor is the medical function unique to psychiatrists. Neurologists are using it for treatment of dementias. Nurse practitioners and clinical pharmacists (doctors of pharmacy) do evaluations and administer medications (medical functions). Usually, they perform these functions under supervision of a physician, but often, in fact, the supervision exists only on paper. Indeed, there are some studies which indicate that some clinical pharmacists choose psychoactive medications more appropriately than do some psychiatrists (Biles, 1983).

If neither the educational functions nor the medical functions are unique to psychiatry, how can psychiatrists hope to define the scope of the profession? There is one function unique to the psychiatrist that can help them know who they are. This function is a good working acquaintance with *both* models. Psychiatry's unique function should be the ability to respond appropriately to people whose mental condition elicits compassion in the context of existential anxiety regardless of which model is triggered. Because psychiatrists are drawn from the ranks of those who have gone to medical school, they will have a medical orientation. The profession probably should (and probably will) center around this model. They do not have to fret about it. As more and more physiological processes and medical responses are discovered, coming from the medical tradition, psychiatrists will learn them. However, to abandon the functions based on the educational model would be to destroy uniqueness, and this would jeopardize the future of the profession (Brodie, 1983).

The scope of psychiatry is not to be defined by fruitless squabbles about whether clusters of mental characteristics are *products of mental illness,* a matter that is beyond the area of psychiatric expertise. Instead, it should be defined by increasing the predictive expertise of its practitioners so that they may respond flexibly and knowledgeably to those people who come for help.

REFERENCES

Adams v. Weinberger, 548 F.2d 239 (1977).

Adler, D. A. (1981). The medical model and psychiatry's tasks. *Hospital and Community Psychiatry, 12,* 387–392.

Akiskal, H. S. (1981). Subaffective disorders: Dysthymic, cyclothymic, and bipolar II disorder in the "borderline" realm. *Psychiatric Clinics of North America, 4,* 25–46.

Alexander, F. G. & Staub, H. (1956). *The criminal, the judge, and the public: A psychological analysis* (rev. ed.). Glencoe, IL: Free Press.

Almond, R., Kenniston, K., & Boltax, S. (1968). The value system of a milieu therapy unit. *Archives of General Psychiatry, 19,* 545–561.

Amarillo, J. (1979). Insanity—guilty but mentally ill—diminished capacity: An aggregate approach to madness. *John Marshall Journal of Practice and Procedure, 12,* 351–382.

American Law Institute (1955). *Model penal code,* tentative draft number 4.

American Law Institute (1962). *Model penal code.*

American Psychiatric Association (1983). Guidelines for legislation on the psychiatric hospitalization of adults. Washington, DC: American Psychiatric Association.

Andreason, N. C., Olsen, A., Dennert, J. W., & Smith, M. R. (1982). Ventricular enlargement in schizophrenia: Relationship to positive and negative symptoms. *American Journal of Psychiatry, 139,* 293–302.

Applebaum, P. S. & Gutheil, T. G. (1980a). Drug refusal: A study of psychiatric inpatients. *American Journal of Psychiatry, 137,* 347–352.

Applebaum, P. S. & Gutheil, T. G. (1980b). Rotting with their rights on: Constitutional theory and clinical reality in drug refusal by psychiatric patients. *Bulletin of the American Academy of Psychiatry and the Law, 8,* 306–315.

Applebaum, P. S. & Gutheil, T. G. (1981). The right to refuse treatment: The real issue is quality care. *Bulletin of the American Academy of Psychiatry and the Law, 9,* 199–202.

Arens, R. (1974). *Insanity defense.* New York: Philosophical Library.

Astrachan, B. M., Levinson, D. J., & Adler, D. A. (1976). The impact of national health insurance on the tasks and practice of psychiatry. *Archives of General Psychiatry, 33,* 785–794.

Ayllon, D. T. & Azrin, N. H. (1965). The measurement and reinforcement of behavior of psychotics. *Journal of the Experimental Analysis of Behavior, 8,* 357–383.

Bakken, C. T. (1970). Counselling services and related operations from a legal viewpoint. In P. T. Galligher & G. E. Demos (Eds.), *The counselling center in higher education.* Springfield, IL: C C Thomas.

Balint, M. (1964). *The doctor, the patient and the illness.* London: Pitman.

Beaver, R. J. (1982). Custody quagmire: Some psychological dilemmas. *Journal of Psychiatry and Law, 10,* 309–326.

Becker, H. S. (1963). *Outsiders: Studies in the sociology of deviance.* New York: Free Press.

Biles, J. A. (1983). The doctor of pharmacy. *Journal of the American Medical Association, 249,* 1157–1160.

Binswanger, L. (1963). The case of Lola Voss. In J. Needleman, *Being-in-the-world: Selected papers of Ludwig Binswanger* (E. Angel, Trans.). New York: Basic Books. (Original work published 1949).

Birnbaum, M. (1960). The right to treatment. *American Bar Association Journal, 45,* 499–505.

Bitner, E. (1967). Police discretion in the emergency apprehension of mentally ill persons. *Social Problems, 14,* 278–292.

Black, D. (1970). Production of crime rates. *American Sociological Review, 35* 735–748.

Bloch, S. & Reddaway, P. (1977). *Psychiatric terror.* New York: Basic Books.

Blocker v. United States, 274 F.2d 572 (1959).

Blocker v. United States, 288 F.2d 853 (1961).

Bodenheimer, E. (1974). *Jurisprudence: The philosophy and method of the law* (rev. ed.). Cambridge: Harvard University Press.

Bolton v. Harris, 395 F.2d 642 (1968).

Bowring v. Godwin, 551 F.2d 44 (1977).

Boydston, J. A. (1980). Malingering. In H. I. Kaplan, A. M. Freedman, & B. J. Sadock (Eds.), *Comprehensive textbook of psychiatry III.* Baltimore: Williams and Wilkins.

Brakel, S. & Rock, R. (1971). *The mentally disabled and the law.* Chicago: University of Chicago Press.

Brickman, P., Rabinowitz, V. C., Karuza, J., Coates, D., Cohn, E., & Kidder, L. (1982). Models of helping and coping. *American Psychologist, 37,* 368–384.

Brodd, C. D. 1952. Ethics and the history of philosophy. London: Routledge and Kegan Paul.

Brodie, H. K. (1983). Psychiatry—its locus and future. *American Journal of Psychiatry, 140,* 965–968.

Bukovsky, V. (1977). Forward. In S. Bloch & P. Reddaway, *Psychiatric terror.* New York: Basic Books.

Bukovsky, V. & Gluzman, S. (1974). A manual of psychiatry for dissenters. In S. Bloch & P. Reddaway, *Psychiatric terror.* New York: Basic Books.

Bursten, B. (1973a). *The manipulator: A psychoanalytic view.* New Haven: Yale University Press.

Bursten, B. (1973b). Decision-making in the hospital community. *Archives of General Psychiatry, 29,* 732–735.

Bursten, B. (1974, February). Psychiatric "expertise" and social values. *Current Medical Dialogue.*

Bursten, B. (1979a). Psychiatry and the rhetoric of models. *American Journal of Psychiatry, 136,* 661–666.

Bursten, B. (1979b). Voluntariness of waiver of Fifth Amendment rights. *Bulletin of the American Academy of Psychiatry and the Law, 7,* 352–362.

Bursten, B. (1980). "Medical responsibility" in institutional settings. *American Journal of Psychiatry, 133,* 1071–1074.

Bursten, B. (1981). Isolated violence to the loved one. *Bulletin of the American Academy of Psychiatry and the Law, 9,* 116–127.

Bursten, B. (1982a). The psychiatrist-witness and legal guilt. *American Journal of Psychiatry, 139,* 784–788.

Bursten, B. (1982b). Narcissistic personalities in DSM III. *Comprehensive Psychiatry, 23,* 409–420.

Bursten, B., Fontana, A. F., Dowds, B. N., & Geach, B. (1980). Ward polity and therapeutic outcome: II. ratings of patient behavior. *Hospital and Community Psychiatry, 31,* 33–37.

Bursten, B. & Geach, B. (1976). Ward polity and therapeutic outcome: I. review of patients' records. *Journal of Nervous and Mental Disease, 163,* 414–419.

Cameron, D. (1969). Nonmedical judgement in medical matters. *Georgetown Law Journal, 57,* 716–733.

Cantor, N. L. (1973). A patient's decision to decline life-saving medical treatment: Bodily integrity vs. the preservation of life. *Rutgers Law Review, 26* 228–264.

Carnahan, W. A. (Ed.). (1978). *The insanity defense in New York.* Albany: State Department of Mental Hygiene.

Carroll, B. J., Feinberg, M., & Greden, J. F. (1981). A specific laboratory test for the diagnosis of melancholia. *Archives of General Psychiatry, 38,* 15–22.

Carter v. United States, 252 F.2d 608 (1957).

Cassell, E. J. (1976). *The healer's art.* Philadelphia: J. B. Lippencott.

Chessler, P. (1972). *Women and madness.* Garden City, NY: Doubleday.

Cloninger, C. R., Reich, T., & Guze, S. B. (1975). The multifactorial model of disease transmission: Sex differences in the familial transmission of sociopathy (antisocial personality). *American Journal of Psychiatry, 127,* 11–22.

Comment. (1964). Manic depressive held incompetent to contract despite ability to understand transaction. *New York University Law Review, 39,* 356–363.

Criss, M. S. W., & Racine, D. R. (1980). Impact of change in legal standard for those adjudicated not guilty by reason of insanity. *Bulletin of the American Academy of Psychiatry and the Law, 8,* 261–271.

Dandridge v. Williams, 397 U.S. 471 (1970).

Davidson, H. (1965). *Forensic psychiatry.* New York: Ronald Press.

Davis v. Hubbard, 506 F. Supp. 915 (1980).

Dershowitz, A. M. (1969, February). The psychiatrist's power in civil commitment: A knife that cuts both ways. *Psychology Today,* 43–47.

Developments in the Law (1974). Civil commitment. *Harvard Law Review,* 1065–1192.

Diagnostic and Statistical Manual of Mental Health Disorders I (DSM I). (1952). Washington, DC: American Psychiatry Association.

DSM II. (1968). Washington, DC: American Psychiatry Association.

DSM III. (1980). Washington, DC: American Psychiatry Association.

Diamond, B. L. (1962). From M'Naughten to Currens and beyond. *California Law Review, 50,* 189–205.

Dix, G. E. (1981). Realism and drug refusal: A reply to Applebaum and Gutheil. *Bulletin of the American Academy of Psychiatry and the Law, 9,* 180–200.

Dressel v. Califano, 558 F.2d 504 (1977).

Dumont, M. P. (1968). *The absurd healer.* New York: Science House.

Durham v. United States, 214 F.2d 862 (1954).

Eckerhart v. Henley, 475 F. Supp. 908 (1979).

Edwards, R. B. (1969). *Freedom, responsibility and obligation.* Hague: Martinns Nijhoff.

Engel, G. L. (1960). A unified concept of health and disease. *Perspectives in Biology and Medicine, 3,* 459–485.

Engel, G. L. (1977). The need for a new medical model: A challenge for biomedicine. *Science, 196,* 129–136.

Enthoven, A. C. (1980). *Health plan: The only practical solution to the soaring cost of medical care.* Reading, MA: Addison-Wesley.

Estelle v. Gamble, 49 U.S. 97 (1976).

Faber v. Sweet Style Mfg. Co., 40 Misc. 2d 212 (1963).

Fabrega, H. (1972). Concepts of disease: Logical features and social implications. *Perspectives in Biology and Medicine, 15,* 583–616.

Farnsworth, D. (1966). *Psychiatry, education and the young adult.* Springfield, IL: C C Thomas.

Faulkner, L. R., Bloom, J. D., & Kundahl-Stanley, K. (1982). Effects of a new involuntary commitment law: Expectations and reality. *Bulletin of the American Academy of Psychiatry and the Law, 10,* 249–259.

Feeley, M. M. (1976). The concept of laws in the social science: A critique and notes on an expanded view. *Law and Society Review, 10,* 497–523.

Feigl, H. (1967). The "mental" and the "physical." In H. Feigl, G. Maxwell, & M. Scriven (Eds.), *Concepts, theories, and the mind-body problem.* Minneapolis: University of Minnesota Press.

Feinstein, A. R. (1968). Clinical epidemiology: The identification rates of diseases. *Annuals of Internal Medicine, 69,* 1032–1061.

Feldman, W. S. (1981). Episodic cerebral dysfunction: A defense in legal limbo. *Journal of Psychiatry and Law, 9,* 193–201.

Finlay v. Finlay, 148 N.E. 624 (1925).

Forst, M. L. (1978). *Civil commitment and social control.* Lexington, MA: Lexington Books.

Frances, A. (1980). The DSM personality disorders section: A commentary. *American Journal of Psychiatry, 137,* 1050–1054.

Frank, J. D. (1971). Therapeutic factors in psychotherapy. *American Journal of Psychotherapy, 25,* 350–361.

Freidson, E. (1970). *Profession of medicine: A study of the sociology of applied knowledge.* New York: Dodd Mead and Company.

Freud, S. (1914). Remembering, repeating and working through. *The Standard Edition of the Complete Psychological Works of Sigmund Freud* (Stand. Ed.), volume 12 (James Strachey, Trans.). London: Hogarth.

Freud, S. (1915). The unconscious. *Stand. Ed,* volume 14.

Frued, S. (1923). The ego and the id. *Stand. Ed,* volume 19.

Fromm-Reichman, F. (1950). *Principles of intensive psychotherapy.* Chicago: University of Chicago Press.

Galach'yan, A. G. (1968). Soviet psychiatry. In A. Kiev (Ed.), *Psychiatry in the communist world.* New York: Science House.

Galper, J. (1973). Personal politics and psychoanalysis. *Social Policy, 4,* 35–44.

Galston, W. A. (1980). *Justice and the human good.* Chicago: University of Chicago Press.

Gaughn, L. D. & LaRue, L. H. (1978). The right of a mental patient to refuse antipsychotic drugs in an institution. *Law and Psychological Review, 4,* 43–85.

Ginsberg v. New York, 390 U.S. 629, 1967.

Gobert, J. J. & Cohen, N. P. (1981). *Rights of prisoners.* Colorado Springs: Shepards McGraw Hill.

Goin, J. & Goin, M. K. (1981). *Changing the body.* Baltimore: Williams and Wilkins.

Goldstein, A. S. (1967). *The insanity defense.* New Haven: Yale University Press.

Goldstein, J., Freud, A., & Solnit, A. J. (1979). *Before the best interests of the child.* New York: Free Press.

Goldstein, J. & Katz, J. (1963). Abolish the "insanity defense"—why not? *Yale Law Journal, 72,* 853–876.

Goldzband, M. (1982). *Consulting in child custody.* Lexington, MA: Lexington Books.

Gordon, G. A. (1966). *Role theory and illness: A sociological perspective.* New Haven: College and University Press.

Gotshalk, D. W. (1968). *Structure and reality: A study of first principles.* New York: Greenwood Press.

Graham, J. R. (1977). *The MMPI: A practical guide.* New York: Oxford University Press.

Grannucci, A. F. (1969). "Nor cruel and unusual punishment inflicted": The original meaning. *California Law Review, 57,* 839–865.

Green, M. D. (1940). Public policies underlying the law of mental incompetency. *Michigan Law Review, 38,* 1189–1221.

Greenberg, L. M., Deem, M. A., & McMahon, S. (1972). Effects of dextroamphetamine, chlorpromazine, and hydroyzine on behavior and performance in hyperactive children. *American Journal of Psychiatry, 129,* 532–539.

Group for the Advancement of Psychiatry (GAP). (1954). *Criminal responsibility and psychiatric expert testimony.* Topeka: Group for the Advancement of Psychiatry.

GAP. (1957). *The role of psychiatrists in colleges and universities* (rev. ed.). New York: Group for the Advancement of Psychiatry.

GAP. (1957). *The role of psychiatrists in colleges and universities* (rev. ed.). New York: Group for the Advancement of Psychiatry.

GAP (1977). *Psychiatry and sex psychopath legislation: The 30's to the 80's.* New York: Group for the Advancement of Psychiatry.

GAP. (1980). *New trends in child custody determination.* New York: Harcourt Brace Javanovich.

Guttmacher, M. S. (1968). *The role of psychiatry in law.* Springfield, IL: C C Thomas.

Hackett, T. P. (1977). The psychiatrist in the mainstream or on the banks of medicine? *American Journal of Psychiatry, 134,* 432–434.

Halleck, S. L. (1967). *Psychiatry and the dilemmas of crime.* Berkeley: University of California Press.

Halleck, S. L. (1974). Legal and ethical aspects of behavior control. *American Journal of Psychiatry, 131,* 381–385.

Halleck, S. L. (1980). *Law in the practice of psychiatry.* New York: Plenum.

Halleck, S. L. (1971). *The politics of therapy.* New York: Science House.

Hampshire, S. (1965). *Freedom of mind.* New York: Harper & Row.

Hansen, C. A. & Plotkin, R. (1977). Brief submitted to U.S. Court of Appeals, First Circuit. Okin v. Rogers. *Mental Disability Law Report, 2,* 43–52.

Harper, F. V. & Kime, P. M. (1934). The duty to control the conduct of another. *Yale Law Journal, 43,* 886–905.

Hart, H. M. (1958). The aims of the criminal law. *Law and Contemporary Problems, 23,* 401–441.

Hartmann, H. (1960). *Psychoanalysis and moral values.* New York: International University Press.

Henry, W. E., Sims, T. H., & Spray, S. L. (1971). *The fifth profession.* San Francisco: Jossey-Bass.

Hermes, T. (1971). On radical therapy. *Radical Therapist, 1,* 2.

Heston, L. (1966). Psychiatric disorders in foster home reared children of schizophrenic mothers. *British Journal of Psychiatry, 112,* 809–825.

Hohfeld, W. N. (1919). *Fundamental legal conceptions.* New Haven: Yale University Press.

Hopt v. People, 104 U.S. 631 (1881).

Humphrey v. Cady, 405 U.S. 504 (1972).

Ingraham v. Wright, 430 U.S. 651 (1977).

In re Ballay, 462 F.2d 648 (1973).

In re Osborne, 294 A.2d 372 (1972).

Jahoda, M. (1958). *Current concepts of positive mental health.* New York: Basic Books.

Jernigan, T. & Katz, L. (1981). *Normal adult variation on computerized C T measures: Comparison with measures from clinical groups.* Presented at the Ninth Annual Meeting of the International Neuropsychology Society, Atlanta, GA.

Joint Committee on Mental Illness and Mental Health. (1961). *Action for mental health.* New York: Basic Books.

Jones v. United States, Sup. Ct. #81-5196, June 29, 1983.

Jones, M. (1953). *The therapeutic community.* New York: Basic Books.

Kaimowitz v. Department of Mental Health. (1973). Reported in *Mental Disability Law Report, 1,* 147.

Karasu, T. B. (1977). Psychotherapies: An overview. *American Journal of Psychiatry, 134,* 851–863.

Karasu, T. B. (1980). The ethics of psychotherapy. *American Journal of Psychiatry,* 1502–1512.

Kelsen, H. (1973). What is justice? In H. Kelsen, *Essays in legal and moral philosophy* (P. Heath, Trans.). Boston: D. Reidel. Original work published 1953)

Kety, S. S., Rosenthal, D., Wender, P. H., & Shulsinger, F. (1968). Mental illness in the biological and adoptive families of adopted schizophrenics. In D. Rosenthal and S. Kety. *Transmission of schizophrenia.* Oxford: Pergamon.

Kittrie, N. N. (1971). *The right to be different: Deviance and enforced therapy.* Baltimore: John Hopkins.

Kornhuber, H. H. (1974). Cerebral cortex, cerebellum and basal ganglia: An introduction to their motor functions. In F. O. Schmidt & F. G. Worden (Eds.), *The neurosciences: Third study program.* Cambridge: MIT Press.

Kowalski, L. J. (1970). Contracts—competency to contract of mentally ill person who understands transaction but is unable to control conduct. *Wayne Law Review, 16,* 1188–1196.

Kunnes, (1970). Psychiatry: Instrument of the ruling class. *Radical Therapist, 1,* 4.

Kupfer, D. J., Foster, F. G., & Coble, P. A. (1978). The application of EEG sleep for the differential diagnosis of affective disorders. *American Journal of Psychiatry, 135,* 69–74.

Lake v. Cameron, 364 F.2d 657 (1966).

Langer, S. (1962). *Philosophy in a new key.* New York: Mentor Books.

Langsley, D. (1980, November, 21). Viewpoint: A commentary by APA's president. *Psychiatric News.*

Lasch, C. (1976, February 22). Sacrificing Freud. *New York Times Magazine,* 90–103.

Lemere, F. & Greenwald, C. T. (1943). Ratio of voluntary enlistment to induction in the various types of neuropsychiatric disorders. *American Journal of Psychiatry, 100,* 312–315.

Levine, D. S. & Willner, S. G. (1976, February). The cost of mental illness. *Mental Health Statistical Note 125.* National Institute of Mental Health, Division of Biometry and Epidemiology.

Levine, R. J. (1978). Forward: The traditional medical model. In M. G. Miller, *Mental illness and the problem of boundaries.* Washington, DC: Medicine in the Public Interest.

Liebman, L. (1976). The definition of disability in social security and supplemental income: Drawing the bounds of social welfare estates. *Harvard Law Review, 89,* 833–867.

Livermore, J. M., Malmquist, C. P., & Meehl, P. E. (1968). Justification for civil commitment. *University of Pennsylvania Law Review, 117,* 75–96.

London, P. (1969). *Behavior control.* New York: Harper & Row.

Ludwig, A. M. & Othmer, E. (1977). The medical basis for psychiatry. *American Journal of Psychiatry, 134,* 1087–1092.

Lykken, D. T. (1979). The detection of deception. *Psychological Bulletin, 86,* 47–53.

Macklin, R. (1982). *Mind and morality: The ethics of behavior control.* Englewood Cliffs, NJ: Prentice-Hall.

MacNamara, D. E. J. & Sagarin, E. (1977). *Sex, crime, and the law.* New York: Free Press.

Maher v. Roe, 432 U.S. 464 (1977).

Mandler, G. & Kessen, W. (1974). The appearance of free will. In S. C. Brown (Ed.), *Philosophy of psychology.* London: Macmillan.

Mannhein, K. (1952). *Essays on the sociology of knowledge.* Paul Kecskmeti (Ed.). London: Routledge and Kegan Paul.

Marcuse, H. (1964). *One-dimensional man.* Boston: Beacon.

Maxmen, J. S., Tucker, G. J., & LeBow, M.D. (1974). Rational hospital psychiatry: the reactive environment. New York: Bruner/Mazel.

May, R. (1939). *The art of counselling.* New York: Whitmore & Stone.

McCormick, H. L. (1983). *Social security claims procedures.* St. Paul: West.

McDonald v. United States, 312 F.2d 847 (1962).

Mechanic, D. (1962). The concept of illness behavior. *Journal of Chronic Diseases, 15,* 189–194.

Mechanic, D. (1980). *Mental health and social policy.* Englewood Cliffs, NJ: Prentice-Hall.

Meldon, A. I. (1961). *Free action.* New York: Humanities Press.

Menninger, K. A. (1968). *The crime of punishment.* New York: Viking Press.

Menninger, W. C. (1952). Therapeutic methods in a psychiatric hospital. *Journal of the American Medical Association, 99,* 538–542.

Meyer v. Nebraska, 262 U.S. 390 (1923).

Miller, F. W. (1969). *Prosecution: The decision to charge a suspect with a crime.* Boston: Little, Brown & Company.

Minirth, F. B. (1977). *Christian psychiatry.* Old Tappan, NJ: Fleming H. Revell.

Mlyniec, W. J. (1977). The child advocate in private custody disputes: A role in search of a standard. *Journal of Family Law, 16,* 1–18.

M'Naughten Case. (1843). 10 Clark & Fin 200.

Monroe, R. R. (1978). *Brain dysfunction in aggressive criminals.* Lexington, MA: Lexington Books.

Nixon, R. E. (1964). Psychological normality in the years of youth. *Teachers Collegiate Review, 66,* 71–79.

O'Connor v. Donaldson, 423 U.S. 563 (1975).

Offer, D. & Sabshin, M. (1980). Normality. In H. I. Kaplan, A. M. Freedman, & B. J. Sadock. *Comprehensive textbook of psychiatry III.* Baltimore: Williams & Wilkins.

Olmstead v. United States, 277 U.S. 438 (1928).

Osborne v. Cohen, 409 F.2d 37 (1969).

Oster, A. M. (1965). Custody proceedings: A study of vague and indefinite standards. *Journal of Family Law, 5,* 21–38.

Overholser, W. (1962). Criminal responsibility: A psychiatrist's viewpoint. *American Bar Association Journal, 48,* 528–531.

Packard, E. P. W. (1973). *Modern persecution or insane asylums unvelied* (reprint). New York: Arno Press. (Original work published 1875)

Packer, H. L. (1968). *The limits of the criminal sanction.* Stanford, Stanford University Press.

Parsons, T. (1951). *The social system.* Glencoe, IL: Free Press.

Parsons v. State, 81 Ala. 577 (1887).

Pearlman, S. (1968). College mental health. In M. Siege (Ed.), *The counselling of college students.*

People v. Gorshen, 51 Cal.2d 716 (1959).

Perkins, R. M. (1939). A rationale of mens rea. *Harvard Law Review, 52,* 905–928.

Pierce v. Society of Sisters, 268 U.S. 510 (1925).

Pinneke v. Preisser, 623 F.2d 546 (1980).

Podlesny, J. A. & Raskin, D. C. (1977). Physiological measures and the detection of deception. *Psychological Bulletin, 84,* 782–794.

Popper, K. & Eccles, J. C. (1977). *The self and its brain.* New York: Springer.

Posner, R. A. (1981). *The economics of justice.* Cambridge: Harvard University Press.

Powell v. Texas, 302 U.S. 514 (1968).

Pribaum, K. H. (1971). *Languages of the brain: Experimental paradoxes and principles in neuropsychology.* Englewood Cliffs, NJ: Prentice-Hall.

Printing and Numerical Registration Co. v. Sampson, 19 Eq. 462 (1875).

Prochaska v. Brinegar, 251 Iowa 834 (1960).

Rand, A. (1965). *The virtue of selfishness.* New York: New American Library.

Reich, W. (1983, January 30). The world of Soviet psychiatry. *New York Times Magazine.*

Rennie v Klein, 653 F.2d 836 (1981).

Restatement (Second) of Contracts. (1973).

Rhodes v. United States, 282 F.2d 59 (1960).

Riese, W. (1953). *The conception of disease: Its history, its versions, and its nature.* New York: Philosophical Library.

Robbins, L. L. (1980). The hospital as a therapeutic community. In H. I. Kaplan, A. M. Freedman, & B. J. Saddock (Eds.), *Comprehensive textbook of psychiatry III.* Baltimore: Williams & Wilkins.

Robitscher, J. B. (1968). Tests of criminal responsibility: New rules and old problems. *Land & Water Review, 3,* 158–176.

Robitscher, J. B. (1980). *The powers of psychiatry.* Boston: Houghton Mifflin.

Roche, P. Q. (1955). Criminality and mental illness: Two faces of the same coin. *University of Chicago Law Review, 22,* 320–324.

Roche, P. Q. (1956). Durham and the problem of communications. *Temple Law Quarterly, 29,* 264–270.

Rock, R. S., Jacobson, M. A., & Janapaul, R. M. (1968). *Hospitalization and discharge of the mentally ill.* Chicago: University of Chicago Press.

Rogers v. Okin, 634 F.2d 650 (1980).

Roman, M. & Haddad, W. (1978). *The disposable parent.* New York: Holt, Rinehart & Winston.

Roth, L. H., Meisel, A., & Lidz, C. W. (1977). Tests of competency to consent to treatment. *American Journal of Psychiatry, 134,* 279–284.

Runions, J. E. (1975). Toward a Christian psychiatry. *Journal of the Christian Medical Society, 6,* 13–19.

Rychlak, J. F. (1973). *Introduction to personality and psychotherapy.* Boston: Houghton-Mifflin.

Ryle, G. (1949). *The concept of mind.* London: Hutchenson.

Santosky v. Kramer, 455 U.S. 745 (1982).

Schafer, R. (1978). *Language and insight.* New Haven: Yale University Press.

Scheff, T. T. (1966). *Being mentally ill.* Chicago: Aldine.

Scholendorf v. Society of New York Hospitals, 105 N.E. 92 (1914).

Schmidt, W. C., Miller, K. S., Bell, W. G., & New, B. E. (1981). *Public guardianship and the elderly.* Cambridge: Ballinger.

Schrag, R. & Divasky, D. (1975). *The myth of the hyperactive child.* New York: Pantheon.

Schwartz, R. A. (1974). Psychiatry's drift away from medicine. *American Journal of Psychiatry, 131,* 129–133.

Selzer, M. L. (1960). The "happy college student" myth: Psychiatric implications. *Archives of General Psychiatry, 2,* 131–136.

Shah, S. A. (1975). Dangerousness and civil commitment of the mentally ill: Some public policy considerations. *American Journal of Psychiatry, 132,* 501–505.

Siegler, M. & Osmond, H. (1974). *Models of madness, models of medicine.* New York: Macmillan.

Sigerist, H. E. (1941). *Medicine and human welfare.* New Haven: Yale University Press.

Simon, R. (1967). *The jury and the defense of insanity.* Boston: Little Brown.

Sinclair v. State, 161 Miss 142 (1931).

Slovenko, R. (1973). *Psychiatry and law.* Boston: Little, Brown and Co.

Smart, J. J. C. (1961). Free-will, praise and blame. *Mind, 70,* 291–306.

Smith v. Califano, 637 F.2d 968 (1981).

Spicer v. Williamson, 132 S.E. 291 (1926).

State v. Jones, 50 N.H. 369 (1871).

State v. Pike, 49 N.H. 399 (1870).

Steadman, J. H., Keitner, L., Braff, J., & Arranites, T. M. (1983). Factors associated with a successful insanity plea. *American Journal of Psychiatry, 140,* 401–405.

Stewart Machine Co. v. Davis, 201 U.S. 548 (1937).

Stoddard, F. J., Altman, H. C., Sheldon, M., Senger, H., & Van Buskirk, D. (1983). Psychiatric benefits and insurance regulations in Massachusetts: A national model? *American Journal of Psychiatry, 140,* 327–331.

Stone, A. A. (1976). *Mental health and the law: A system in transition.* New York: Jacob Aronson.

Stone, A. A. (1981). The right to refuse treatment. *Archives of General Psychiatry, 38,* 358–362.

Szasz, T. S. (1961). *The myth of mental illness.* New York: Hoeber-Harper.

Szasz, T. S. (1963). *Law, liberty and psychiatry: An inquiry into the social uses* of mental health practices. New York: Macmillan.

Szasz, T. S. (1965). *Psychiatric justice.* New York: Macmillan.

Szasz, T. S. (1970). *Ideology and insanity.* New York: Doubleday Anchor.

Szucko, J. J & Kleinmutz, B. (1981). Statistical versus clinical lie detection. *American Psychologist, 36,* 488–496.

Tancredi, L. R. & Slaby, A. E. (1977). *Ethical policy in mental health care: The Goals of psychiatric intervention.* New York: Prodist/William Heinemann Medical Books.

Task Panel on Community Mental Health Centers Assessment. (1978). *Task panel* report to the President's Commission on Mental Health, 2. Washington, DC: U.S. Government Printing Office.

Task Panel on Legal and Ethical Issues. (1978). *Task panel reports submitted to the President's Commission on Mental Health, 2.* Washington, DC: U.S. Government Printing Office.

Task Panel on the Nature and Scope of the Problem. (1978). *Task panel report submitted to the President's Commission on Mental Health, 2.* Washington, DC: U.S. Government Printing Office.

Tater v. Tater, 120 S.W. 2d 203 (1938).

Thorne v. Weinberger, 530 F.2d 203 (1976).

Torrey, E. F. (1974). *The death of psychiatry.* Radner, PA: Chilton.

Trop v. Dulles, 356 U.S. 862 (1958).

Trunnell, T. L. (1976). Johnnie and Susie, don't cry: Mommie and daddy aren't really that way. *Bulletin of the American Academy of Psychiatry and the Law, 4,* 120–126.

United States v. Brawner, 471 F.2d 969 (1972).

United States v. Currens, 290 F.2d 751 (1961).

United States v. Freed, 401 U.S. 601 (1971).

United States v. Freeman, 357 F.2d 606 (1966).

United States v. Green, 26 F. Cas. 30 (1824).

United States v. Leach, Crim. No. 450–457 O. D.C. (1957).

Vanaguanas, S. & Elliot, J. F. (1980). *Administration of police organization.* Boston: Allyn & Bacon.

Van den Berghe, P. L. (1977). Bridging the paradigms: Biology and the social sciences. In M. S. Gregory, A. Silvers, & D. Sutch (Eds.), *Sociobiology and human nature.* San Francisco: Jossey-Bass.

Vorenberg, E. W. & Vorenberg, J. (1973). Early diversion from the criminal justice system: Practice in search of a theory. In L. E. Oblin (Ed.), *Prisoners in America.* Englewood Cliffs, NJ: Prentice-Hall.

Washington v. United States, 390 F.2d 444 (1967).

Wertham, F. (1955). Psychoauthoritarianism and the law. *University of Chicago Law Review, 22,* 336–338.

Wexler, D. B. (1973). Token and taboo: Behavior modification, token economies, and the law. *California Law Review, 61,* 81–104.

Whitley, J. V. (1979). Mental health of college students. *Journal of the American College Health Association, 28,* 92–95.

Wilson, E. O. (1975). *Sociobiology: The new synthesis.* Cambridge: Harvard University Press.

Wing, J. K. (1978). *Reasoning about madness.* London: Fakenham & Reading.

Wyatt v. Stickney, 344 F. Supp. 373 (1972).

Zilboorg, G. (1968). *The psychology of the criminal act and punishment.* New York: Greenwood.

Index

A

Adams v Weinberger, 154
Adjustment disorder, 175–177, 202, 229
Adler, D A, 20, 235
Advocacy, 169, 181–184
Akiskal, H S, 35
Alcoholism, 25–26, 77, 90, 102, 111, 152, 154,
    155, 166, 220
Alexander, F G, 108–109
Almond, R, 186
Amarillo, J, 94, 106
American Psychiatric Association, 23, 24, 26,
    110–112, 122, 133
Amnesia, 85–86, 92, 228
Andreasen, N C, 90–91
Anorexia nervosa, 186
Antisocial personality, 23–25, 109, 111, 112,
    126–127
Anxiety disorder, 38, 87, 156, 163, 198, 205,
    229
Applebaum, P S, 131, 132
Arens, R, 109, 111
Astrachan, B M, 20
Ayllon, D T, 186
Azrin, N H, 186

B

Bakken, C T, 146
Balint, M, 173
Bazelon, D, 4, 5, 66, 70, 94, 121
Beaver, R J, 195
Becker, H S, 6
Biles, J A, 237
Binswanger, L, 225
Biofeedback, 235–236
Birnbaum, M, 159

Bitner, E, 98
Black, D, 97
Bloch, S, 7, 126–130
Blocker v U.S. (1959), 25
Blocker v U.S. (1961), 109
Blood pressure, 224
Bodenheimer, E, 70
Bolton v Harris, 210
Borderline personality, 3, 23, 127, 194, 211,
    230
Bowring v Godwin, 162
Boydston, J A, 84
Brakel, S, 137, 203
Brandeis, L E, 115
Brickman, P, 232–234, 236
Broad, C D, 40
Brodie, H K, 238
Bukovsky, V, 125, 127–130, 208
Burger, W, 109
Bursten, B, 15, 21, 41, 53, 74, 76, 102, 132,
    142, 169, 186, 187, 188, 205, 214, 224,
    237

C

Caffeinism, 235
Cameron, D, 164
Cantor, N L, 132
Cardozo, B N, 71, 192
Carnahan, W A, 110
Carroll, B J, 90
Carter v U.S., 45
Cassell, E J, 222–225
Catatonia, 186
Chessler, P, 8, 180
Child,
    best interests of, 192–193, 196
    custody, 14, 87, 169, 189–197

Choosing, 20, 39–43, 47–49, 52–58, 60–62, 63, 69, 71, 76, 78–81, 84, 105, 108, 119, 143, 167–170, 182, 191, 202, 221, 232–234
Claims, 115–116, 142–143, 159, 160
Cloninger, C R, 35
Coercion, 167–169, 172–173, 177, 180, 186–190, 196
Cognition, 51–55, 57, 70, 75, 77, 79, 82, 91, 106–109, 111, 112, 116–117, 122, 133, 138–139, 144
Cohen, N P, 162
Commitment, 12, 71–73, 99, 101, 118–130, 133–135, 160, 169, 182, 185, 197, 206–208, 210–213
Compulsive personality, 11
Contracts, 12, 72, 142–145, 190
Conversion disorder, 83, 87, 158, 228–229
Criss, M S W, 95
Cruel and unusual punishment, 104–105, 130–131, 160
Cyclothymic personality, 8, 35

D

Dandridge v Williams, 162
Davidson, H, 88
Davis v Hubbard, 214
Defensiveness, 177, 178–179
Delirium, 136, 228
Dementia, 79–80, 152, 228, 229, 237
Dependent personality, 176
Depression, 29–30, 31, 35, 53, 57, 90, 137, 148, 149, 163, 175–176, 205, 224, 228
Dershowitz, A M, 121
Determinism, 20, 28, 32–34, 39–43, 45–49, 53, 56, 60, 62, 63, 65, 69, 71, 72, 74, 76, 78–81, 84, 108–109, 112, 140–141, 154, 158, 163, 167–168, 170
Deviance, 6, 8, 20, 26, 30, 35, 37, 68, 69, 97, 159, 190, 220–221, 232–236
Diamond, B L, 64, 110
Disability, 14–15, 143, 150–157
Discipline, 15, 16–19, 198, 206–216, 232
    in general medical hospital, 17, 215–216
    in psychiatric hospital, 18–19, 132, 134, 206–208, 213–214
Dissociative disorder, 111
Divosky, D, 18
Dix, G E, 118

Dressel v Califano, 152
Drug abuse, 35, 77, 90, 102, 111, 152, 229
Dumont, M P, 180
Durham v U.S., 4–5, 9, 45, 47, 108–109
Duval, A, 23–25, 43, 64

E

Eccles, J C, 36, 54
Eckerhart v Henley, 159
Education, 169, 232–238
Edwards, R B, 232
Ego strength, 42
Elliot, J F, 97
Emotion, 51, 53–55, 64–70, 71, 75, 77, 79, 82, 109, 117, 122, 133, 139
Employment, 16–17, 71, 215
Engle, G L, 21, 222, 226
Enthoven, A C, 216
Estelle v Gamble, 160
Existential anxiety, 224–238

F

Faber v Sweet Style Mfg. Co, 144
Fabrega, H, 222
Farnsworth, D, 146
Faulkner, L R, 123
Feely, M M, 72
Feigl, H, 36
Feinstein, A R, 222–223
Feldman, W S, 54
Finlay v Finlay, 192
Forst, M L, 203
Frances, A, 38
Frank, J D, 173
Free will, 20, 28, 39–43, 48–49, 71, 105, 110, 224
Freidson, E, 27
Freud, S, 19–20, 50, 53, 178
Fromm-Reichman, F, 179

G

Galach'yan, A G, 125
Galper, J, 180
Galston, W A, 217
Gaughn, L D, 131
Geach, B, 132, 187

Ginsberg v. New York, 191
Gluzman, S, 127–130, 208
Gobert, J J, 162
Goin, J, 140
Goin, M K, 140
Goldstein, A, 12, 65–66, 95, 103, 106
Goldstein, J, 105, 189, 193
Goldzband, M, 189
Gordon, G A, 60
Gotshalk, D W, 36
Graham, J R, 89
Grannucci, A E, 104
Green, M D, 143
Greenberg, L M, 18
Greenwald, C T, 6
Group for the Advancement of Psychiatry, 42–43, 147, 189, 192, 202, 203, 205
Guthiel, T G, 131, 132
Guttmacher, M S, 108

H

Hackett, T P, 234
Haddad, W, 192
Halleck, S L, 121, 140, 174, 181, 201
Hampshire, S, 40, 48
Hangmen, 129, 208–209
Hansen, C A, 130
Harper, F V, 73
Hart, H M, 65, 104
Hartmann, H, 74, 181
Henry, W E, 232
Hermes, T, 8
Heston, L, 35
Histrionic personality, 176
Hohfeld, W N, 142
Homosexuality, 25–26, 173–174
Hopt u People, 77
Hospitals,
    general medical,
        discipline in, 17, 215–216
        treatment refusal in, 13
    psychiatric,
        commitment to, 12, 71–73, 99, 101, 118–130, 133–135, 160, 169, 182, 185, 197, 206–208, 210–213
        discipline in, 18–19, 132, 134, 206–208, 213–214
        milieu, 132, 169, 178, 184–188

Humphrey u Cady, 118, 202
Hypochondriasis, 228–229
Hypoparathyroidism, 33–34, 35

I

Identity viewpoint, 36–37, 223
Illness, definition of, 26–44, 221–226
Immune rights, 115–116, 142, 159, 160
Impulsivity, 51, 53, 229
Incompetence, 116–117, 138
    to contract, 112, 143–145
    to manage affairs, 137–140
    to refuse general medical treatment, 13, 136–137, 140–141
    to refuse psychiatric hospitalization, 118–125
    to refuse psychiatric treatment, 12, 13, 133–135, 160, 212–213
Inexperience, 19–20, 97, 220–238
Informed consent, 117, 130, 144
Ingraham u Wright, 130
In re Ballay, 118
In re Osborne, 135
Insanity defense, 4–5, 10, 24–25, 64–66, 73, 77, 79–82, 94–114, 124–130, 150, 154, 197, 200, 202–205, 210–213
Interaction viewpoint, 36, 37, 223–224, 227, 235
Intermittent explosive disorder, 78, 111

J

Jahoda, M, 27
Jernigan, T, 91
Jessel, M R, 143
Jones, M, 181
Jones u U.S., 213

K

Kaimowitz u Department of Mental Health, 130
Karasu, T B, 172, 236
Katz, J, 105
Katz, L, 91
Kelsen, H, 66
Kessen, W, 40
Kety, S S, 35
Kime, P M, 73

Kittrie, N N, 8, 118, 120, 203
Kleinmutz, B, 90
Kleptomania, 54, 200–202, 229
Kornhuber, H H, 54
Kowalski, L J, 144
Kunnes, R, 8
Kupfer, D J, 90

L

Lake u Cameron, 121
Langer, S, 36
Langsley, D, 124
La Rue, T H, 131
Lasch, C, 182
Laziness, 7, 14–15, 19
Lemere, C T, 6
Levine, D S, 161, 162
Levine, R, 222–224
Libertarianism, 40–43, 48–49, 63, 65, 69, 71,
    72, 74, 78–81, 84, 112, 154, 167–168, 170
Liebman, L, 150, 157
Liver disease, 224
Livermore, J M, 118
London, P, 168–169, 172, 173, 180
Ludwig, A M, 20, 234
Lykken, D T, 90

M

McCormick, H L, 151
McDonald u U.S., 113
Macklin, R, 167
MacNamara, D E J, 203
Maher u Roe, 162
Malingering, 14–15, 83–93, 102, 146, 152, 155,
    157, 158, 159, 168
Mandler, G, 40
Mania, 31, 35, 53, 54, 57, 144, 152, 163–164,
    175, 222, 228
Manipulation, 7, 14–15, 19, 169, 205, 216, 232
Mannheim, K, 21
Marcuse, H, 130, 171
Maxmen, J S, 185, 186
May, R, 19–20
Mechanic, D, 58, 161, 163, 167
Melden, A I, 48
Menninger, K, 140
Menninger, W, 184

Mens rea, 104, 105
Meyer u Nebraska, 191
Miller, F W, 84, 200
Minirth, F B, 10
Minnesota Multiphasic Personality
    Inventory, 89
Mlyniec, W J, 191, 192
M'Naughten's Case, 106–108, 109, 111
Monroe, R R, 54

N

Narcissistic personality, 13, 113, 190, 194, 211
Naturalistic explanations, 11, 20, 28, 32–34,
    43, 169, 224
Nixon, R E, 148
Normality, 6

O

O'Connor u Donaldson, 159
Offer, D, 27
Olmstead u U.S., 115
Osborne u Cohen, 154
Osmond, H, 20, 234
Oster, A M, 189
Othmer, E, 20, 234
Overholser, W, 23–25, 43, 64

P

Packard, E P W, 206
Packer, H L, 105
Pain, psychogenic, 27, 83, 152, 155, 158,
    228–229
Paranoid disorder, 102, 126, 228
Paranoid personality, 28
Parens patriae, 118–120, 122, 131–132, 133,
    136, 144, 191, 192
Parson, T, 27, 60
Parsons u State, 108
Pearlman, S, 146, 147
People u Gorshen, 110
Perkins, R M, 104
Personal injury, 87, 143, 157–158
Phillistines, 129, 208–209
Pierce u Society of Sisters, 191
Pinneke u Preisser, 163
Plotkin, R, 130

Pneumonia, 58
Podlesny, J A, 89
Police officers, 9, 10, 94–103, 112, 126, 200
Police power, 118–120, 132, 133
Political dissenters,
    general, 31–32, 180
    Soviet Union, 7–8, 125–130
    United States, 6–7, 121, 126, 208–209
Polygraph, 89–90
Popper, K, 36, 54
Posner, R A, 218
Postconcussive syndrome, 158
Posttraumatic stress disorder, 15, 47, 84, 158
Pound, E, 209
Powell u Texas, 154
Praiseworthy behavior, 6, 7–9, 30, 126, 179,
    220
Prediction, ix, 32, 140–141, 147–148, 163, 174,
    182, 195, 202, 212–213, 238
Pribram, K H, 54
Printing and Numerical Registration Co. u
    Sampson, 143
Prisons,
    hospitals as alternatives to, 24, 185, 202,
        210–211
    psychiatric treatment in, 160–161, 162
Prochaska u Brinegar, 118
Psychiatric treatment,
    induction into, 11, 173–175, 176
    refusal of, 12, 130–137
    request for, 143, 159–166
Psychiatry,
    domain of, ix, 20–22, 220–238
    political use of, 6–8, 31–32, 121, 125–130,
        180, 208–209
    radical, 8
Psychotherapy, 11, 15, 19–20, 30, 131, 169,
    172–181, 184, 188, 196

R

Racine, D R, 95
Rand, A, 72
Raskin, D C, 90
Reddaway, P, 7, 126–130
Reich, W, 129
Relaxation training, 236
Rennie u Klein, 12, 130
Rhodes u U.S., 110

Riese, W, 222, 223, 226
Right to treatment, 159
Robbins, L L, 186
Robitscher, J B, 8, 14, 25, 26, 42, 115, 171, 180,
    209
Roche, P Q, 47
Rock, R S, 9, 137, 203
Rogers u Okin, 12, 119, 136
Roman, M, 192
Roth, L H, 117
Runions, J E, 10
Rychlak, J F, 19
Ryle, G, 48

S

Sabshin, M, 27
Sagarin, E, 203
Santosky u Kramer, 191
Schafer, R, 40, 48, 49
Scheff, T T, 38
Schizoid personality, 211
Schizophrenia, 29, 35, 38, 53, 56, 60, 77, 84,
    89, 104, 117, 126, 128, 129, 148–149,
    152, 156, 163–164, 220
Schizotypal personality, 35, 90–91, 230
Schmidt, W C, 137–138
Scholendorf u Society of New York Hospital, 130
Schrag, R, 18
Schwartz, R A, 236
Selzer, M L, 148
Sex offenders, 54, 152, 202–205
Shah, S A, 120
Siegler, M, 20, 234, 236
Sigerist, H E, 226
Simon, R J, 111
Sin, 7, 10–11, 220–238
Sinclair u State, 104–105
Slaby, A E, 217
Slovenko, R, 107, 109
Smart, J J C, 6
Smith u Califano, 154
Social Security, 14–15, 143, 150–157, 216
Sociobiology, 67–68, 70, 225
Somatization disorder, 88
Soviet Union, 7–8, 125–130
Spicer u Williams, 160
State u Jones, 50
State u Pike, 5

Staub, H, 108–109

Steadman, J H, 113

Stoddard, F J, 217

Stone, A A, 105, 120, 121–122, 130

Story, J, 192

Student mental health, 14, 17–18,
　　145–150

Sufficient mental illness, 75–80, 98, 124, 153,
　　161, 164, 177, 179, 180, 182–183, 188,
　　194, 230

Szasz, T S, 8, 15, 29, 40, 115, 130, 171, 199,
　　206, 209

Szucko, J J, 90

T

Tancredi, L R, 217

Tater u Tater, 192

Third party payment, 21, 159–166, 198,
　　216–219

Thorne u Weinberger, 152

Threshold mental illness, 76–80, 87, 91, 92,
　　111–112, 113, 126, 128, 129, 153

Torrey, E F, 20, 29, 226

Transduction,
　　as coercion, 177
　　in advocacy, 182–183
　　in child custody cases, 193, 195
　　in commitment proceedings, 122,
　　　　124–125, 128, 129, 208
　　in decision making, 159
　　in definition of psychiatry, 231
　　in employment cases, 218
　　in guardianship cases, 139
　　in incompetence decisions, 116
　　in insanity defense, 79–82, 111, 112,
　　　　113
　　in personal injury cases, 158
　　in police custody situations, 97, 99,
　　　　103
　　in requests for treatment, 164–165
　　in sex offender cases, 204
　　in social security decisions, 156–157
　　in student requests, 149

on general medical wards, 137

Trop u Dulles, 105

Trunnell, T L, 195

Tuberculosis, 28

U

Undesirable behavior, 6, 7, 26, 30–32, 35, 143,
　　169–197, 224, 226

Unpleasant behavior, 15–18, 97, 102, 232

Unwise behavior, 7, 11–14, 97, 115–141,
　　220–238

Urge, 53–55, 75, 77, 79, 82, 91, 108, 109, 117,
　　122, 133, 139, 144, 204

U.S. u Brawner, 5, 66, 94

U.S. u Currens, 107

U.S. u Freed, 104

U.S. u Freeman, 77

U.S. u Green, 191, 192

U.S. u Leach, 24

V

Values, 167–197

Vanagunas, S, 97

Van den Berghe, P L, 68

Vorenberg, E W, 200

Vorenberg, J, 200

W

Warren, E, 105

Washington u U.S., 81, 112

Wertham, F, 47

Wexler, D B, 187

Whitley, J L, 147

Wilner, S G, 161, 162

Wilson, E O, 68

Wing, J K, 27, 38, 39

Wyatt u Stickney, 187

Z

Zilboorg, G, 140